A Clinical Guide To Crowns And Other Extra-Coronal Restorations

A Clinical Guide To Crowns And Other Extra-Coronal Restorations

R W Wassell
Senior Lecturer in Restorative Dentistry, The School of Dental Sciences, Newcastle upon Tyne

A W G Walls
Professor of Restorative Dentistry, The School of Dental Sciences, Newcastle upon Tyne

J G Steele
Senior Lecturer in Restorative Dentistry, The School of Dental Sciences, Newcastle upon Tyne

F S A Nohl
Consultant in Restorative Dentistry, Newcastle Dental Hospital

D J Jacobs
Consultant in Restorative Dentistry, Newcastle Dental Hospital

J M Whitworth
Senior Lecturer in Restorative Dentistry, The School of Dental Sciences, Newcastle upon Tyne

E R Smart
Lecturer in Restorative Dentistry, The School of Dental Sciences, Newcastle upon Tyne

G St George
Specialist Registrar in Restorative Dentistry, Eastman Dental Hospital, London

F M Blair
Consultant in Restorative Dentistry, Birmingham Dental Hospital

R P Ingledew
Senior Dentist, Boots Dental Care, Maidenhead

D Barker
Higher Specialist Trainee in Restorative Dentistry, Newcastle Dental Hospital

2002

Published by the British Dental Association
64 Wimpole Street, London, W1G 8YS

Acknowledgement

The authors would like to acknowledge Alan Walker for his excellent line diagrams and his unfailing good humour.

ISBN 0 904588 73 4

Printed and bound by Dennis Barber Limited, **Lowestoft, Suffolk**

Contents

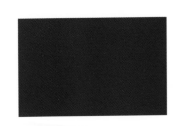

Crowns and other extra-coronal restorations: Introduction

R. W. Wassell[1] J. G. Steele[2] and A. W. G.Walls[3]

This series of articles is aimed at anybody who places crowns and other extra-coronal restorations (ie veneers and adhesive onlays or 'shims') on individual teeth. We hope that everyone from experienced practitioners to undergraduate students may find something of value. The aim of this series is to give guidance, based on available scientific evidence where possible, towards the provision of high quality restorations.

Treatment planning issues and materials choices feature at least as strongly as technique description.

We have concentrated on single tooth restorations, but all of the principles described also apply to more complex multiple restorations, including fixed bridges. However, we have not specifically covered replacement of missing teeth with bridges or implants. Replacement of teeth involves consideration of a range of additional issues and treatment planning decisions, whilst an entirely different set of technical rules are required for the consideration of implants. These will be left for other authors to address.

Where possible, we refer to published scientific evidence. Admittedly, randomly controlled clinical trials and systematic reviews are much scarcer in dentistry than in medicine. Consequently, much evidence is based on the experience of clinicians, or on laboratory or theoretical considerations. This does not necessarily devalue existing practices, but it does make it more difficult to make objective choices about treatment planning, materials or techniques. We have therefore tried to be honest when our advice stems solely from experience or theory.

The series consists of 13 individual articles, each of which should be able to stand alone. Each article will start with the specific learning objectives we hope to meet. In a series like this it is impossible to explore every technique or material ever described, this would make for very heavy reading and very dull writing. We hope though that these articles should enable the reader to evaluate his or her own practices against a set of fundamental principles.

CONTENT OF THE SERIES
A series of 13 Articles covering the following:

1. Changing patterns and the need for quality
2. Materials considerations
3. Pre-operative assessment
4. Endodontic considerations
5. Jaw registration and articulator selection
6. Aesthetic control
7. Cores for teeth with vital pulps
8. Preparations for full veneer crowns
9. Provisional restorations
10. Impression materials and technique
11. Try-in and cementation of crowns
12. Porcelain veneers
13. Resin bonded metal restorations

[1]*Senior Lecturer in Restorative Dentistry, [2]Senior Lecturer in Restorative Dentistry, [3]Professor of Restorative Dentistry, Department of Restorative Dentistry, The Dental School, Framlington Place, Newcastle upon Tyne NE2 4BW
*Correspondence to: R. W. Wassell
E-mail: r.w.wassell@ncl.ac.uk

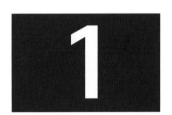

IN BRIEF

- Crown provision has seen an enormous increase over the past three decades. In the UK around 1 million teeth are fitted with crowns every year, many of these requiring complex additional treatment prior to crown placement
- Around 15% of NHS dental spending annually is on crown provision and maintenance, so the total cost is very large
- The pressures on dentists to produce high quality restorations is probably increasing and will not diminish
- There are few data on the quality or longevity of restorations placed
- Technological advances have changed the way we are able to practice over recent decades, and further developments will open up new possibilities

Crowns and other extra-coronal restorations: Changing patterns and the need for quality

J. G. Steele[1] R. W. Wassell[2] and A. W. G. Walls[3]

This series of articles is aimed at anybody who places crowns and other extra-coronal restorations (ie veneers and shims) on individual teeth. We hope that everyone from experienced practitioners to undergraduate students may find something of value. Whoever reads them, we would ask to do so with an open mind. We have tried not to be dogmatic, and the techniques and materials described are not the only ones available, but are the ones which accord with the principles we describe.

[1]*Senior Lecturer in Restorative Dentistry,
[2]Senior Lecturer in Restorative Dentistry,
[3]Professor of Restorative Dentistry,
Department of Restorative Dentistry,
The Dental School, Framlington Place,
Newcastle upon Tyne NE2 4BW
*Correspondence to: J. G. Steele
E-mail: jimmy.steele@ncl.ac.uk

Our aim in these articles is, by working from a sound theoretical base, to try to give the reader the background to pick the best treatment options from the wide, and continuously changing, range available. Technical issues are important and will be addressed, but there is a need to recognise that the provision of extra-coronal restorations is more than just cutting a shape which is free of undercuts, on to which something can be cemented. Cutting a preparation and cementing a restoration are relatively easy. Cutting a preparation and cementing a restoration which will last for many years without any further damage to the dental tissues is a different matter. Treatment planning issues and materials choices will occupy a greater part of this series of articles than the technicalities of tooth preparation.

We have concentrated on single tooth restorations, but all of the principles described also apply to more complex multiple restorations, including fixed bridges. However, we have not specifically covered replacement of missing teeth with bridges or implants. Replacement of teeth involves consideration of a range of additional issues and treatment planning decisions, whilst an entirely different set of technical rules are required for the consideration of implants. These will be left for future authors to address.

In an ideal world we would have been able to draw on the conclusions of full systematic reviews of the literature, based on randomised controlled clinical trials. Such an approach is widely used in many areas of medicine and allows objective assessment of the available techniques, drugs or materials. Few such reviews are available in this area of dentistry though, probably because the raw material from which

they are derived, namely randomised controlled clinical trials, are themselves so sparse. Where possible, we have tried to support what we write with appropriate previously published scientific evidence, but good quality evidence is scarce and much of what has been written in the past is based on the experience of clinicians, or on theoretical considerations. This does not necessarily

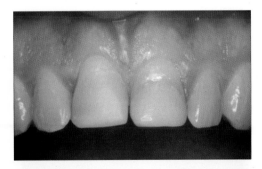

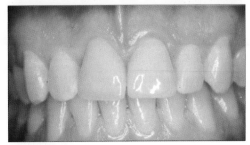

Fig. 1a and 1b. The provision of good quality crowns or alternative adhesive restorations can result in a tremendous improvement in oral health for the patient as well as being a fulfilling experience for the dentist. Despite being a relatively minor procedure, this patient's aesthetics and confidence were improved enormously by the provision of these anterior dentine bonded crowns

A guide to crowns

Fig. 2 A series of radiographs taken over a five year period showing how the provision of crowns can be detrimental to oral health where the treatment is ill thought out and, in this case, poorly executed. This is a graphic illustration of 'the need for quality'

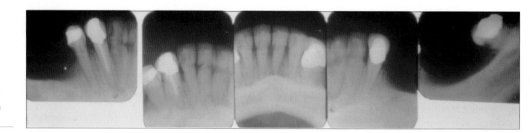

Fig. 2a Initial presentation revealed crowns on lower anterior teeth with early root caries on several teeth

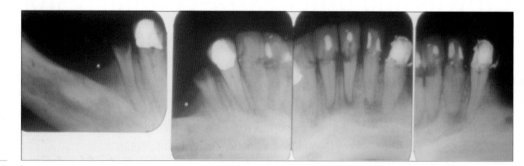

Fig. 2b Treatment is planned and started but the caries has progressed and periapical pathology quickly becomes apparent. Root treatment is started on affected teeth, without dealing with the root caries and its causes

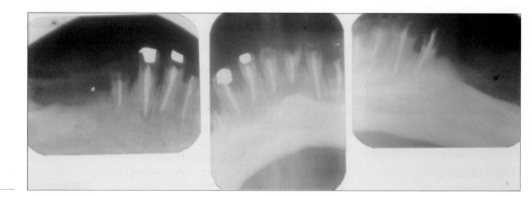

Fig. 2c Root treatment continues apace but with little attention to coronal seal

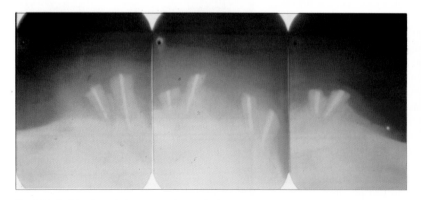

Fig. 2d A decision is made to progress to overdentures

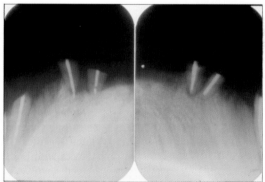

Fig. 2e Periodontal attachment loss and periapical pathology render overdenture abutments useless

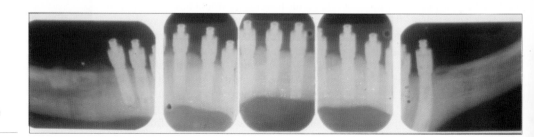

Fig. 2f A successful outcome, but a little late in the day

devalue existing practices, but it does make it more difficult to make objective choices about treatment planning, materials or techniques. We have tried to identify where there is and where there is not strong evidence to support what we write, but inevitably we have often had to write from experience or theory.

The series consists of 13 individual articles, each of which should be able to stand alone. For each of these we will set, at the start of the paper, the specific learning objectives which we hope to meet. In a series like this it is impossible to explore every technique or material ever described, this would make for very heavy reading and very dull writing. We hope though that these articles should enable the reader to evaluate his or her own practices against a set of fundamental principles.

The rest of this article will present some background data which illustrate the health benefits, the health problems, the scale and the cost of crown provision, and the potential for technological change to help us to improve oral health.

BACKGROUND: THE NEED FOR QUALITY

Crowns and oral health

As we progress in the new millennium, a rich blend of improving technology, better oral health, a strengthening scientific base and the timeless ability to employ fine manual skills and artistry are making it increasingly possible, and enjoyable, for the dentist to deliver good quality restorations. Moreover, it is also increasingly possible to do this with the minimum of damage to the dental tissues.

The health benefits of providing high quality restorations are essential, substantial and long lasting. Current concepts of health include positive aspects of quality of life; self esteem and the ability to undertake daily activities, such as eating, speaking and socialising, comfortably and without embarrassment. It is here that restorative dental care has a major impact on health. Even in a simple case, such as that in Figure 1a, where an incisal tip has fractured and the composite repair is functional but dull, lifeless and unsightly in the eyes of the patient, the pre-treatment restoration can be a cause of embarrassment. Well executed restorations could (and did, see Fig. 1b) make a substantial positive impact on this individual's well being. In a dentition extensively broken down by years of disease and wear the functional and aesthetic disability can be much greater and the benefit more dramatic. It is true that poorly executed treatment may have the opposite effect. Figure 2 shows a series of radiographs of a patient where crowns have been poorly conceived, ill-planned and carelessly executed. The case is as graphic an illustration of the need for both good planning and skilful execution as it is possible to find, and we will be using this case to illustrate a number of specific points in a later article.

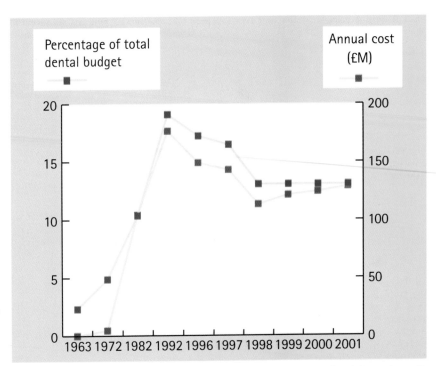

Fig. 3 The cost of overall crown provision under the National Health Service for adults aged over 18 years, 1963 to 1995/96 (figures for cost not taking into account annual inflation) (Note: The scale on the x-axis is non-linear)

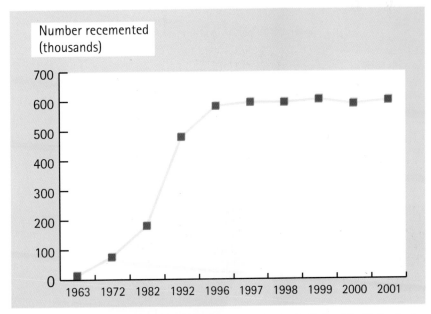

Fig. 4 The total number of crowns (in thousands) recemented under the National Health Service for adults aged over 18 years, 1963–1995/96 (Note: The scale on the x-axis is non-linear)

Historical trends

The number of crowns placed by dentists in Europe and North America is vast and in many countries the volume has been increasing year on year. In England and Wales, where data are available from the National Health Service (NHS), the number of treatments showed a rapid increase over the past 30–40 years with the cost peaking at nearly £180M in 1991/1992 (Fig. 3).[1-5] It reduced significantly in the early 1990s when some dentists moved out of NHS practice following contractual changes, and then very markedly in 1997 when porcelain fused to metal restorations on molar teeth were removed from

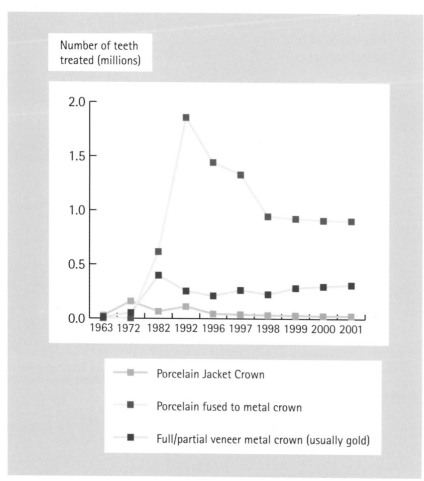

Number of teeth treated (millions)

- ■ Porcelain Jacket Crown
- ■ Porcelain fused to metal crown
- ■ Full/partial veneer metal crown (usually gold)

Fig. 5 The total number of crowns of different types (all metal, porcelain fused to metal and all porcelain) provided under the National Health Service for adults aged over 18 years, 1963–1995/96 (Note: The scale on the x-axis is non-linear)

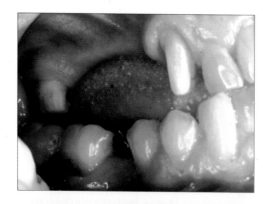

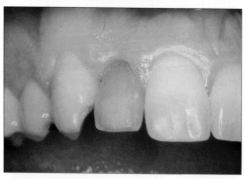

Fig. 6a and 6b Adhesive dentistry has much to commend it. Contrast the destructive preparation for conventional porcelain fused to metal restoration (4a) with the much more conservative preparation for a porcelain veneer (4b)

the list of permitted items. Despite the reduction, the sums spent are still vast: around £142M in 2000-2001 for crowns alone, but £6M for veneers, £11.5M for large onlays (having undergone a very sharp rise since 1997) and £33.5M for bridges. Around a third of the dentate adult population have at least one artificial crown, and amongst adults now in their 50s and 60s, half have a crown. Those with crowns have around three per head on average.[6] These figures are derived from the *1998 UK Adult Dental Health Survey* and show a marked increase from the situation a decade earlier. Data from other countries are less easily available, but what data there are suggest that trends in Western Europe and North America are broadly similar.

The dental and demographic trends in the population will ensure that the need for full coverage and other extra-coronal restorations will not diminish in the foreseeable future. In addition to the need to maintain and replace existing crowns, there is a tidal wave of heavily restored teeth in the middle-aged group in many western countries which resulted from treatment of higher levels of caries in the 1950s, 60s and 70s.[6] These heavily restored teeth are now getting old. As the restorations in them age they will need to be replaced, and as they are replaced they will get larger. The number of cases where there has been extensive loss of tooth tissue, and therefore where full coverage restorations may be indicated, looks unlikely to diminish. It may even increase. Furthermore, the need for such restorations will tend to be concentrated towards the older end of the age spectrum, providing an additional challenge for the clinician. At the same time increasingly litigious consumers will demand high quality restorations, and may be prepared to recover their costs through the courts if their treatment is ill-conceived or poorly executed. The pressures on practising dentists to produce high quality restorative dentistry has never-been higher, and will not reduce.

Quality issues

Despite the vast number of crowns placed and the need for high quality, we know very little indeed about the performance of these restorations. Even simple data on the longevity of crowns, and the rate of loss or replacement are limited. Research findings are often difficult to interpret because of variability in the selection criteria and treatment techniques used. Certainly, the number of crowns which are dislodged and require to be recemented is large in the UK; well over half a million crowns are recemented every year under the NHS. This figure rose rapidly in the 1980s and 90s reflecting the increase in overall crown provision(Fig. 4).[1–5] But, crowns which fall out are only one manifestation of failure. Others include those which become carious, periodontally compromised or in which the pulps become inflamed or necrotic as a result of the treatment provided. Evidence for the long-term effects of crown preparation on vital teeth is very sparse indeed. There are estimates of the damage to pulp vitality which occurs following tooth reduction for crowns and bridges. This indicates that anything from 1–15% of teeth lose vitality after preparation, with two of the three studies cited here approaching the higher end of the range.[7-9] For various reasons these estimates may not be representative of typical adult populations, but they do indicate that irreversible pulp damage is likely to be a substantial problem. There are very few useful quantitative data on other forms of failure. In these articles we have tried to use the limited evidence available to identify and then to address the reasons for failure.

Technological solutions

Technological advances over the past 30 years have offered many potential solutions to some of these problems, and have in turn played their part in changing treatment patterns as well. The traditional boundaries between routine and advanced restorative work have become blurred as new techniques and materials have proliferated, so much so that we found it difficult to decide on a title for this series of articles. All metal and all porcelain restorations have largely given way to porcelain fused to metal restorations (Fig. 5 shows data for the UK National Health Service),[1-5] but changes in porcelain technology are starting to provide improved all-porcelain alternatives again, though it may be some time before their use becomes widespread. Looking beyond this, it is possible to envisage a greater place for composite resins as an alternative to porcelains in future years. However, it is the rapid development of adhesive technology, particularly where bonding to dentine is concerned, that has provided the greatest potential for change and the most exciting possibilities. Above all, preparations can be

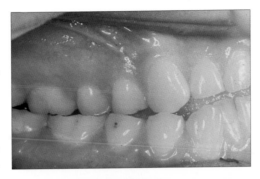

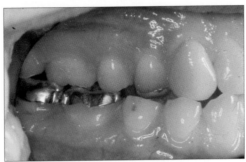

Fig. 7a and 7b With the spectrum of restorations now available, some cases are best treated with a combination of conventional and adhesive approaches

made much less destructive and are often quicker to cut (Figs 6a and 6b). For all their attractions though, adhesive restorations create their own problems. Provisional restorations are difficult to make, and the final restoration is often awkward to adjust and to cement. They are highly technique sensitive, requiring additional skills and care if they are to be successful.

In this series we will attempt to outline a set of principles for the provision both of conventional and adhesive restorations (Figs 7a and 7b) with the aim of improving oral health.

1   Dental Practice Board. *Digest of Statistics 1995-2001.* Part 1-Detailed analysis of GDS treatment outcomes. DPB, Eastbourne. Data for 1996-2001 available at: http://www.bdta-dentistry.org.uk/dentaldata/index.html

2   Dental Practice Board. *Digest of Statistics 1991-92.* Part 1-Detailed analysis of GDS treatment outcomes. DPB, Eastbourne.

3   Dental Estimates Board. *Statistics 1963.* DEB, Eastbourne.

4   Dental Estimates Board. *Annual Report 1972.* DEB, Eastbourne.

5   Dental Estimates Board. *Annual Report 1982.* DEB, Eastbourne.

6   Kelly M, Steele J, Nuttall N, Bradnock G, Morris J, Nunn J, Pine C, Pitts N, Treasure E, White D. *Adult Dental Health Survey: Oral Health in the United Kingdom in 1998.* (2000) London: TSO.

7   Felton D, Madison S, Kanoy E, Kantor M, Maryniuk G. Long term effects of crown preparation on pulp vitality. *J Dent Res* 1989; **68** (special issue):1009. Abstract 1139.

8   Bergenholtz G, Nyman S. Endodontic complications following periodontal and prosthetic treatment of patients with advanced periodontal disease. *J Periodontol* 1984; **55**: 63-68.

9   Reuter J E, Brose M O. Failures in full crown retained dental bridges. *Br Dent J* 1984; **157**: 61-63.

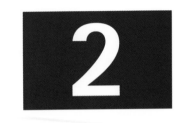

IN BRIEF

- Familiarisation with the broad spectrum of contemporary materials allowing better-informed decisions to be made
- Discovering the factors that influence choice of alloys for indirect metallic restorations
- Knowing the pitfalls of selecting a cheap alloy for cast post and core construction
- Familiarisation with the different types of all ceramic crown and which ones can be used posteriorly
- An awareness of the many different types of metal copings for ceramo-metal restorations
- Consideration of the use of composite crowns for specific clinical situations

Crowns and other extra-coronal restorations: Materials selection

R. W. Wassell[1] A. W. G. Walls[2] and J. G. Steele[3]

Materials selection is the second in the series on crowns and other extra-coronal restorations. Some of us are less than inspired by dental materials science. Nevertheless, many of the things that concern us clinically with crowns and their alternatives are based on material properties. We worry about the strength of the restoration, how well it fits and its aesthetics. We also worry about wear, occlusal control and biocompatibility. Not least of our concerns are dental laboratory charges, which inevitably have to be passed on to the patient.

[1]*Senior Lecturer in Restorative Dentistry,
[2]Professor of Restorative Dentistry,
[3]Senior Lecturer in Restorative Dentistry,
Department of Restorative Dentistry, The Dental School, Framlington Place, Newcastle upon Tyne NE2 4BW
*Correspondence to: R. W. Wassell
E-mail: r.w.wassell@ncl.ac.uk

An understanding of the materials available, their application and limitations will not only help with selection but will allow more effective communication with patients and laboratories. Promotion of such understanding allowing better-informed decisions to be made is in essence the aim of this article.

There are now more materials available than ever before for indirect restorations. These fall under the broad headings of all metal, ceramics, metal-ceramics and resin composites. Cements and cementation, either conventional or adhesive will be considered in later articles. Manufacturers' details are shown at the end of the article.

ALL METAL RESTORATIONS

All metal extra-coronal restorations include crowns, onlays and shims (onlays relying solely on adhesive retention). Cast posts and cores can cause particular difficulties and are considered separately at the end of this section. In the UK as in other countries we are aware that economic pressures are driving the adoption of less expensive alloys. These alloys contain either low concentrations of noble metals or are comprised entirely of base metals.

In this section we consider the various types of alloys and the factors which influence their selection including:

- Cost
- Castability and handling
- Physical properties
- Resin bonding
- Corrosion and tarnish
- Biocompatibility

Gold and palladium alloys

In the 1950s making an alloy selection for a cast metal restoration would simply have entailed choosing an ADA specification high gold alloy, all of which had a greater than 75% gold and platinum content. The soft type I alloy contained most noble metals (83%) with the harder alloys (types II, III and IV) containing an increasing amount of silver and copper. Type I alloy was used for small inlays, type II for larger inlays, type III for crowns and bridges, and type IV for partial denture frameworks.

In the early 1970s the gold price increased four fold resulting in the introduction of less expensive alloys of lower Karat.[1] Palladium, which had been used since the 1930s to produce a cheaper white gold (Au 30%, Pa 10–35%, Ag 35-60%, Cu 6–25%), became the noble constituent of many of the new precious alloys. These alloys include:

- Silver-palladium
- Palladium-silver-gold
- Gold-silver-copper-palladium (with a gold content greater than 40%)
- Palladium-copper
- Palladium-tin

Palladium has a strong whitening effect which means that most of these alloys will have a silvery appearance unless the gold content is greater than 40% and the palladium less than 6%.[2] Unfortunately, both palladium and silver absorb oxygen when molten, which can result in porous castings especially if casting buttons are reused. Also, reducing the gold content lowers the specific gravity (density), which may make casting less reliable than with high gold alloys. This is because less dense alloys have lower kinetic energy during casting which in turn reduces the penetration of molten metal into the mould. Nevertheless, some authorities argue that with ideal conditions almost all commercial alloys result in acceptable castings,[3] but experience indicates that technicians may find such conditions difficult to achieve.

Tarnishing of some alloys is noticeable in certain patients, particularly around the margins of their restorations. This observation is born out by a five-year clinical study comparing two palladium silver alloys to a type III gold alloy.[4] In the UK the National Health Service has encouraged the use of alloys containing only 30% gold. The potential for corrosion problems to result from this change is currently unknown.

Allergies to gold, palladium and platinum are extremely rare.[5] *In-vitro* studies[6] show that high gold alloys have excellent corrosion resistance, which implies that few metal ions are eluted from restorations. Metal ions are eluted more easily from alloys of low noble metal content, including those of copper and silver. Copper ions have been implicated in producing lichenoid reactions.[7] However, lichenoid reactions to metal ions from crowns are not as well described as for amalgam where many lichen planus series show up to a third of patients to be sensitive to mercury salts.[8] This raises the possibility that some cases of lichen planus adjacent to crowns may be linked to the underlying amalgam core. Nevertheless, with current trends to use more easily corrodible casting alloys we should be alert to the possibility of more lichen reactions in the future.

Base metal alloys
Base metal alloys used to make indirect restorations include:

- Nickel-chromium
- Nickel-chromium-beryllium
- Titanium
- 'Progold'

Nickel-chromium alloys
The most commonly used base alloys are nickel-chromium and nickel-chromium-beryllium. Beryllium is added to improve the alloy's physical properties; it is used as a hardener, grain structure refiner and to reduce the alloy's fusion temperature.[9] As a result of health concerns (see below) some alloys contain molybdenum instead of beryllium.[10] All of these alloys have a higher modulus of elasticity than noble alloys. This means that they are more rigid which is helpful in preventing flexion of long span bridges. Rigidity in thin section is necessary for adhesive bridge frameworks and for adhesively retained shims used to restore the palatal surfaces of worn incisors. It is also possible with selected resin adhesives to obtain high bond strengths to the surface of the sandblasted alloy. For instance Nery *et al.*[11] reported a bond strength of 22 Mpa for a nickel chromium alloy bonded to dentine with All Bond 2 (Bisco Inc,

Itasca, USA). A worrying trend, however, is for some laboratories to substitute a precious metal instead of nickel chromium without telling the dentist. Clearly, this could reduce the expected bond strength.[10]

Leaving aside health concerns for a moment, nickel chromium alloys are not without problems. Casting conditions need to be carefully controlled to obtain well fitting restorations and any technician will tell you that these alloys are hard to adjust and difficult to finish. This in turn can be a nuisance clinically when fitting restorations.

Experience of use differs markedly from country to country. In the USA these alloys have had a relatively good press[12,13] and are used for casting crowns and bridges by the majority of laboratories.[9] In the UK these alloys account for only 1% of the crowns provided on the National Health Service. In Sweden, the National Board of Health and Welfare has warned against the use of alloys containing more than 1% nickel,[9] effectively precluding nickel-chromium alloys as they all contain between 62 and 82% nickel.[14]

The health problems are worth exploring in more detail. Many laboratories use non-beryllium containing nickel chromium alloys, as beryllium grindings and casting fumes are extremely hazardous unless controlled by an adequate exhaust and filtration system. Acute problems include conjunctivitis, dermatitis and bronchitis. Chronic beryllium disease may not express itself for several years after exposure.[9] Similarly, nickel can cause technicians dermatological and lung problems with high levels of nickel or nickel compounds being carcinogenic. Tumours include rhabdomyosarcoma, nasopharyngeal and lung carcinomas. Again an effective exhaust system is needed to keep concentrations below recommended levels (Table 1). These levels vary from country to country, but if you are fitting nickel chromium restorations you should ensure adequate aspiration during adjustments.

Nickel is well known to cause contact dermatitis. Current estimates show that between 10–20% of women and 1–2% of men are sensitised to the metal, possibly as a result of wearing nickel containing jewellery.[15] Surprisingly, there have been few reports of patients reacting adversely to nickel containing dental restorations and little evidence that nickel adsorption intra-orally exacerbates existing dermatitis. Nevertheless, there are authorities that counsel dentists against using nickel in those patients known to be sensitive to the metal.[5,14]

Table 1 Nickel and beryllium are toxic. In the UK maximum permitted air levels (in μg.m^{-3}) of nickel for an eight-hour shift have recently been reduced five fold[78] but are still over six times higher than in the USA[9]

	UK	USA
Beryllium	2	2
Nickel	100	15

Titanium

Titanium and its alloys are well known for biocompatibility. Restorations can be either cast or electro-formed. Casting requires high temperatures (1650°C) and a special magnesium investment.[16] Titanium oxidises easily so an argon arc is used to melt the metal and casting performed under vacuum. In 1985, Ida *et al.*[17] reported that the fit of cast titanium crowns was intermediate between those made from a high noble alloy and nickel chromium. Electro-forming was introduced in 1989[18] and involves the milling of a titanium blank by spark erosion. Two year clinical follow-up of electro-formed copings veneered with composite have shown encouraging results.[19]

'Progold'

Do not be misled by alloys such as 'Progold'. Like brass they consist largely of copper and zinc, and tarnish easily.

Cast post and cores

To avoid the post bending or breaking, the alloy chosen should have relatively high hardness, proportional limit and ultimate tensile strength. Occasionally, cost considerations drive the selection of the cheapest alloy, however corrosion and problems with castability should always be born in mind; porosity within a cast post can often result in post fracture with unfortunate consequences and thin posts are more likely to suffer critical porosity than thicker ones.

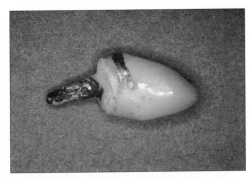

Fig. 1 A bent cast post has resulted in failure (note the failed composite cementation). Proper alloy selection and heat treatment will produce a more rigid casting, capable of resisting distortion from occlusal forces.

It is important to note that many gold alloys used for post and cores can be either soft or hard depending on heat treatment. A soft post will bend (Fig.1) and break more easily under occlusal load than a hard one. Laboratories may unwittingly produce soft posts simply by quenching the hot casting ring to allow the investment to be easily removed. If this is done the casting must be heat-treated according to manufacturer's specifications. The alloy used at our dental hospital (45% Ag, 28.8% Pd, 18.8% Cu, 5% Au, 0.6% Pt) is heat treated at 400°C for 20 minutes. In practice our technicians avoid the need for a separate heat treatment by allowing

the casting ring to bench cool slowly to room temperature.

Some of the alloys used for all metal restorations can also be used for metal-ceramic restorations. However, we will first consider all ceramic restorations.

ALL CERAMIC RESTORATIONS

Dental ceramics, also termed porcelains, have a composite structure consisting of a crystalline phase or phases within a glassy matrix. Dental ceramics consist of oxides, largely of metals and silica, and are essentially inert materials, but we should be aware that they can be attacked by acidulated phosphate fluoride (APF) gel. Clinical experience with all ceramic restorations breaking under occlusal load confirms that these materials are generally susceptible to stress corrosion and slow crack growth.[20]

In 1965 McClean introduced aluminous porcelain.[21] Until then only feldspathic porcelain had been available to make PJCs which although aesthetic was extremely brittle. Many of us would now consider aluminous porcelain as the standard material for PJCs. Nevertheless, despite it being a significant advance and highly aesthetic, aluminous PJCs are still prone to fracture and cannot be recommended as reliable means of restoring posterior teeth.

There are now a bewildering number of porcelain systems on the market and research is continuing to develop materials which are strong, aesthetic and suitable for multiple applications, including crowns, bridges, inlays and onlays. Some materials rely on the production of an opaque, heavily reinforced core over which weaker but more aesthetic layers of porcelain are built eg In-Ceram and AllCeram. Other materials have the strengthening agent dispersed throughout the material e.g. the glass ceramic, Dicor. Details of the strengthening mechanisms are well described elsewhere[22] but all of them rely on having a crystalline phase dispersed within a glassy matrix.

Traditionally, porcelains are classified as high fusing, medium fusing or low fusing but this is not terribly helpful in understanding the increasing number of materials available. Aluminous porcelain PJCs are made simply by sintering (see later) but there are five other methods of making indirect porcelain restorations which together form a useful means of classification:

- Sintered Porcelains
- Glass Infused Ceramics
- Cast Glass Ceramics
- Hot Pressed, Injection Moulded Ceramics
- Machined Glass Ceramics
- Machined Densely Sintered Ceramics

We will first consider some of the materials within this classification and then look at the major clinical factors that influence material choice.

Methods of making indirect porcelain restorations

Sintered porcelains

Sintered porcelains are built up from an aqueous slurry of porcelain particles condensed onto a platinum foil matrix or a refractory die. Sintering occurs at a temperature above the softening point of porcelain whereby the glassy matrix partially melts and the powder particles coalesce. There is volume shrinkage of 30–40%. Porosity can be reduced from 5.6 to 0.56% by vacuum firing.[23] Sintering is the most commonly used technique of making PJCs and veneer restorations with a number of different materials available:

- Aluminous porcelain eg Vitadur-N, Hi-Ceram
- Feldspathic porcelain reinforced with Zirconia fibres eg Mirage II
- Feldspathic porcelain reinforced with leucite eg Optec HSP

Glass infused ceramics

In-Ceram is a glass infused ceramic used for crowns (Fig. 2). It consists of a core containing 90% alumina, which is built up on a refractory die. During firing, at 1150°C for four hours, the die shrinks so that it can be withdrawn from the core. This process (which is also used to manufacture ceramic lavatory pans) is called 'slip-casting'. At this stage the core is a weak, porous structure consisting of partially sintered alumina particles. Strength is conferred by painting a slurry of lanthanum containing glass onto the outside of the core and refiring it. During refiring the molten glass is drawn into the porous structure thus eliminating voids and creating a glass-ceramic composite. The excess glass is ground away and porcelain with a matched coefficient of thermal expansion is built onto the surface. The manufacturers recommend that restorations be cemented with conventional acid base cements.

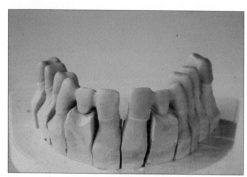

Fig. 2 In–Ceram glass infused alumina cores prior to porcelain application (Courtesy of Vita)

In-Ceram Spinnel is a similar type of material but uses the less hard magnesium spinnel (MgAl$_2$O$_4$) instead of alumina. The material is specifically designed for inlays and onlays. Most recently introduced is In-Ceram Zirconia, which has a very high flexural strength.

A novel material called Techceram has been introduced in the UK, which also relies on having a glass infused core. The core is built of small 'splats' of alumina sprayed from a plasma gun at a rotating refractory die. Again, after glass infusion, the restoration is formed conventionally on the core with a matched sintered porcelain. The company claim a flexural strength as high as for In-Ceram.

Cast glass ceramics

Glass ceramics are polycrystalline solids prepared by the controlled crystallisation of glasses. The best known of these systems, Dicor, is based on mica crystals although there is another, Cerapearl, based on hydroxyapatite and experimental lithia-based materials.[24] A Dicor restoration is made by investing a wax pattern and casting. Heating the reinvested crown for six hours at 1070°C carries out controlled crystallisation, termed 'ceraming'. This causes the Mica to form a strong 'house of cards' structure, which makes fracture propagation equally difficult in all directions. However, a reaction between the mica and the surrounding investment may result in a weakened surface layer, which reduces significantly the overall strength of the material.[25] Characterisation of the crown is achieved by surface glaze. Prior to glazing the material has the appearance of frosted glass.

To overcome the limitations of surface glaze, which are considered in more detail later, a technique of laminating a Dicor coping with feldspathic porcelain has been developed with the intriguing name 'Willi's Glass'.[26] Providing the correct porcelain (Dicor Plus) is used for lamination, the strength of the restoration should not be adversely affected.[27]

Hot pressed, injection moulded ceramics

IPS Empress is a leucite containing porcelain. As with cast glass ceramics the restoration is first waxed-up and invested, however the ingot, which is made of sintered ceramic, is not molten but softened before being pressed into a mould under pressure at 1150°C (Fig. 3). The pressure is maintained for 20 minutes during which time the tetragonal leucite crystals are dispersed throughout the restoration giving a 40% concentration by volume. The shade of the ingot provides the basic shade, which can be modified by either glazing or veneer porcelains. To ensure compatibility with veneer porcelains the ingots have a lower coefficient of thermal expansion (14.9 x 10^{-6}/°C) than those for the glazed material (18 x 10^{-6}/°C). The application of veneer porcelains may require multiple firings that can enhance the strength of the material.[28]

Another material, less well known in the UK is Alceram, which is based on magnesium spinnel. It is important to emphasise that this is a quite different material to the much stronger Procera AllCeram which is mentioned later.

Machined glass ceramics

There are a number of milling systems available for milling ceramic blanks,[29] which may be con-

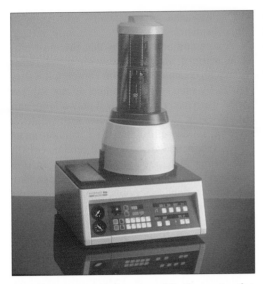

Fig. 3 The press ceramic furnace used for the construction of injection moulded IPS Empress crowns (Courtesy of Ivoclar).

trolled either by computer aided design/computer aided manufacture (CAD/CAM) or mechanically. The best-known CAD/CAM system in the UK is Cerec and the best-known manual system is Celay. Both of these machines were introduced for inlays and onlays, but the original Cerec 1 software gave questionable marginal fit.[30–32] The accuracy of fit is better with Cerec 2[33] and may be improved still further with the recent introduction of Cerec 3.

The ceramic blanks are manufactured to higher levels of strength than can be achieved manually in the dental laboratory. Materials include Dicor MGC, Vita Mark II and Vita Celay; the latter two contain sanidine ($KAlSi_3O_8$) as the crystalline phase. Unfortunately, sanidine makes the ceramic very opaque.[22] A newer material, Corning MGC-F is a tougher material with a higher flexural strength.[34]

Despite the relatively high strength of the ceramic blank, machining may cause weakening through the introduction of surface flaws.[35]

Machined densely sintered ceramics
Procera AllCeram is a densely sintered, high purity alumina core on which low fusing porcelain is built.[36,37] AllCeram cores have some of the highest measurements of flexural strength yet recorded for a commercially available system. Despite this, even stronger materials based on zirconia are being developed.

Interestingly, the cores are made centrally in Sweden or New Jersey, USA. Local dental laboratories scan the dies (Fig. 4) and the information is sent to one of the two centres via the Internet enabling oversized dies to be made. The dies are oversized to compensate for the shrinkage of alumina during sintering. A mixture of alumina and binder is pressed onto the dies under pressure and, before sintering, machined to the required thickness (0.25, 0.4 or 0.6 mm). In this way any small defects caused by machining are eliminated

during sintering. The thicker cores are recommended for posterior teeth and the thinner cores for veneers. The 0.4 mm cores are used for aesthetically critical crowns on anterior teeth and first premolars.

Choice of ceramic system
When faced with the task of evaluating a new or alternative ceramic system you should have a number of questions in mind — as considered under the six headings below.

Should I choose the strongest ceramic?
The flexural strength of ceramics is often quoted (see Table 2 for moduli of rupture), but it is worth pointing out the limitations of such data (see later) before automatically choosing what appears to be the strongest system on the list.

- Fracture toughness and fatigue are also important
- Comparisons between tests may be unreliable [38,39]
- An In-Ceram core, although strong in itself, is weakened by increasing the thickness of overlying ceramic[40]
- Resin cements are an important adjunct to the strength of the finished restoration. This concept has been shown with veneers.[41] A poor bond of resin to tooth or restoration will not enhance the strength of the cemented restoration. Some ceramic cores are smooth internally and resistant to etching with hydrofluoric acid (eg In-Ceram), which prevents effective resin bonding unless specific silanisation techniques are used.[42,43]
- Some ceramic veneers omit the strengthening core and rely mainly on the resin bond to enhance the strength of the comparatively weak veneering ceramic.

How much tooth reduction is needed?
Most systems specify a similar amount of tooth reduction as for a conventional alumi-

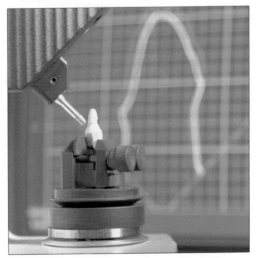

Fig. 4 A die is scanned for a Procera AllCeram coping (outline of scan is in the background), which is made centrally in either Sweden or the USA (Courtesy of Nobel Biocare)

Table 2 Comparative flexural strength data for dental ceramics classified according to technique of restoration production

Crystalline Phase	Example	Flexural Strength (MPa)	Reference
Sintered Porcelains			
Aluminous (Pt foil)	Vitadur-N	123	79
Aluminous (refractory die)	Hi-Ceram	139	79
Leucite reinforced	Optec HSP	104	79
Zirconia based	Mirage II	70	79
Glass Infused Ceramics			
Alumina based	In-Ceram	446	80
Magnesium spinnel	In-Ceram Spinnel	378	80
Zirconia	In-Ceram Zirconia	604	80
Cast Glass Ceramics			
Mica based	Dicor	125	79
Hot Pressed Injection Moulded Ceramics			
Leucite based	IPS Empress	97	80
		160-180	28
Zirconia and Alumina	Alceram	162	81
Machined Glass Ceramics			
Mica based	Dicor MGC	229	80
Sanidine	Vita Mark II	122	80
Machined Densely Sintered Ceramics			
Alumina	Procera AllCeram	687	36

nous PJC; that is a 1 mm shoulder and 1.5 to 2 mm incisal reduction for anterior teeth and 2 mm occlusal reduction for posterior teeth. A 1.2 mm axial reduction is specified for In-Ceram but a much heavier axial preparation is needed (1.5 mm) when Dicor crowns are prescribed for posterior teeth. Many dentists will find this unacceptably destructive of tooth tissue or they simply will not cut it and then wonder why the crown fractures.

Do all ceramic restorations fit well?

The marginal fit of indirect restorations is for many dentists an emotive but inconclusive subject. There is currently no consensus as to what constitutes an unacceptable marginal opening [44] although clinical experience and empirical data suggest 100μm[45] especially where the margin can only be probed.[46] No relationship has been found between size of marginal opening and microleakage,[47] however an open margin will predispose to loss of cement lute, which has implications for secondary caries and periodontal disease.[48]

Most marginal fit data is from *in-vitro* studies where variables are carefully controlled but unfortunately comparisons of crown types are limited and studies cannot be compared because of differences in methodology. Also, measurements can be made difficult by rounding of shoulder ceramic margins. These in-vitro studies generally show mean marginal openings in the 20–80 mm range and while statistically significant differences can be shown between systems[49] the clinical relevance is unclear. However, as already mentioned[1] some of the machined ceramic restorations have much greater discrepancies. Those would certainly be problematic if

the restorations were cemented with conventional cements.

A common perception is that the most reliable margins are achieved with metal rather than with ceramic. Whilst this contention is supported by some studies[49] others do not support it.[50] Clearly technical skill will play a large part in achieving satisfactory results with whatever system is chosen. Comparing ceramo-metal crowns to metal crowns with all ceramic crowns the former generally have better resistance to marginal distortion from repeated firings than the latter, which has implications for some all ceramic systems where the ceramic is applied incrementally.[51] In-Ceram, however, has good resistance to multiple firings.[52]

Will the system be aesthetic?

Although all ceramic restorations have the potential to provide the best aesthetics, aesthetics are material and skill dependent. Obtaining a good result is not simply a matter of colour matching. Translucency, which is determined by the match in reflective indices of the crystalline phase and surrounding matrix, is also important. Better control of colour can be achieved by building it into the substance of the restoration rather than merely relying on surface glaze which may wear thin with time or be removed with adjustments. Some of the systems described above are coloured entirely by surface glazing.

Will the restoration abrade the opposing tooth?

Ceramic has a reputation for causing wear to opposing tooth structure. This is born out by in-vitro studies,[53] and certainly there is a potential for greater wear if ceramic is left rough after occlusal adjustment.[54] It is currently not clear if one type of ceramic is markedly less abrasive than the others, although the mica-glass, Dicor, the machinable glass Vita Mark II and the low fusing ceramics (eg Procera and Duceratin) have shown a trend in this direction.[55,56,57] The situation is complex however; chemicals in foodstuffs (eg cola drink) may affect some low fusing ceramics resulting in them becoming more abrasive and less resistant to wear.[58] Further research is needed before dentists can confidently prescribe ceramic occlusal surfaces with similar abrasivity to gold.

Is the system supported by meaningful clinical studies?

The problem with clinical studies is that they take time. Longevity data at one or two years is of limited use unless it is showing a high failure rate. Also clinical success with anterior crowns can not be extrapolated posteriorly; a 3-year trial of Dicor molar crowns resulted in a failure rate of 64%. With the brittle characteristics of all ceramic restorations, a trial of 5 years is preferable to be confident of future performance. Good data is available for In-Ceram[59,60] and for Procera AllCeram[61] showing fracture levels of less than 1% per year.

Are all ceramic bridges possible?

It is possible to make small anterior bridges with most of these systems, but with the exception of Vita's In-Ceram few manufacturers actively promote this because of the risk of fracture, especially at the connectors. The Procera AllCeram specifies a minimum connector height of 3 mm and a maximum span of 11 mm. Clinical studies are underway but long-term results are not yet available.

Cost?

The cost of high strength ceramic restorations such as In-Ceram, AllCeram and Empress will take into account a laboratory's investment in new equipment and training as well the time taken to make a restoration. In the UK, high strength ceramic crowns are up to £40 to £60 more expensive than an aluminous PJC. These materials can be used on the National Health Service but not without prior approval. If approved, a discretionary fee is awarded which in most cases will not cover the laboratory bill.

METAL–CERAMIC RESTORATIONS

Stress concentrations within PJCs often lead to cracks propagating outwards from the fit surface of the restoration. A comparatively tough metal coping effectively bonded to the ceramic will help stop cracks developing in this way. The first metal copings were cast but other methods of coping construction, including foil and metal composite copings, have since been developed.

Cast copings

Porcelain fused to metal (metal-ceramic) technology was first described in 1956[62] and patented in 1962.[63] Alloys were produced with melting points sufficiently high to resist the firing of porcelain. The first alloys had a high noble metal content of around 98% with iron, indium and tin used for hardening, and to create a superficial oxide layer to which the ceramic could be bonded. The ceramic had to be specially formulated to have a high coefficient of thermal contraction to prevent unwanted stresses being built up between it and the coping on cooling after firing. This was achieved with a ceramic containing 15–25 vol% leucite as its crystalline phase.

With such a high gold content the original alloys were extremely expensive, resulting in many laboratories preferring high palladium low gold alloys – although paradoxically, palladium prices have recently been so high that the high gold alloys are sometimes the more affordable alternative! High palladium alloys have the advantage of having a high modulus of elasticity and are therefore more rigid allowing slightly thinner copings to be made. This rigidity is particularly useful in bridgework where flexion of the pontics under load can result in fracture of the overlying porcelain. The alloy used by our dental hospital contains 78.5% Pa, 6.9% Cu, 5.5% Ga, 4.5% In, 2% Sn, 2% Au. Other alloys also contain either gallium or indium or both to promote chemical bonding to the porcelain.[10]

Some of the alloys already considered under 'all metal restorations' can be used for metal-ceramic copings. These include nickel chromium, nickel chromium beryllium, silver palladium alloys and titanium.

Control of the oxide layer thickness is important to avoid problems of porcelain debonding. Some silver palladium alloys can cause a greenish hue to appear due to diffusion of silver compounds into the porcelain. Titanium oxidises easily and a thick nonadherent oxide layer can form under regular feldspathic porcelains. Thus low fusing porcelains (eg Procera or Duceratin) are used to avoid problems of the oxide layer compromising strength.[64] Porcelain bond strengths to titanium are in any case not as high as with other alloys which may explain the higher risk of metal-ceramic failure seen in a 6-year clinical follow-up.[65]

Low fusing 'hydrothermal' porcelains (Duceram, Duceragold) can also be fused to type IV gold in what is known charmingly as the 'Golden Gate System'. Once again control of the oxide layer is crucial for achieving bonding and good aesthetics.[66] Aesthetics are improved by the underlying gold shining through the porcelain. The major perceived advantage of this system is the potential to limit the number of different alloys used in a patient's mouth.

Cast copings are the most commonly used method of strengthening porcelain and have served us well, but consistently good aesthetics are difficult to achieve because the metal has to be covered by an opaque layer which in turn limits the thickness of an adequate overlying layer of porcelain. However, proper tooth reduction and excellent technical support will largely overcome this problem.

One of the main advantages of cast copings is that the coping can be waxed to create a metal occlusal surface – a facility that is either absent or more difficult to achieve in the following two systems.

Foil copings

In 1976 McClean [67] reported a technique of fusing platinum foil to the fit surface of an aluminous PJC. The foil was made adhesive to the porcelain by electroplating with tin and subsequent oxidisation. The crown was made using two layers of foil with the first layer being removed after firing.[68] Any improvements in compressive strength are controversial with some reports showing a positive effect and others negative.[69] Such differences are explained by variations in test methodology. Other foils have been tried with aluminous porcelain including palladium[70] and gold coated platinum.[71,72] More recently a gold foil reinforced crown has been introduced.[73] The foil of this 'Sunrise Crown' is 50 μm thick and contains gold, platinum and an oxidising element designed to facilitate porcelain bonding. Unlike platinum foil, the gold alloy has too high a coefficient of thermal expansion to be used with aluminous porcelain. Standard metal-ceramic porcelains are used instead. These crowns can fit well[74] but measurements of compressive strength are unimpressive,[73] and, in the absence of clinical trials to the contrary, do not support their use for restoring posterior teeth.

Metal composite copings

The Captek system was developed over a decade ago for producing composite metal frameworks for metal-ceramic crowns, bridges, inlays and onlays (Fig. 5). The technique, which involves the fabrication of a metal composite (Fig. 6) coping (88% Au, 4% Pt, 4% Pa) is comparatively simple but does require some technician training.[75] A metal impregnated wax sheet is adapted over a refractory die, sintered in a porcelain furnace, and the resulting granular structure infused with molten gold. The coping thickness is 250 µm for anterior teeth and 350 µm for posterior teeth. The margins can be thinned down to 50 µm to give a gold micro-margin or a porcelain butt fit produced. Conventional metal-ceramic porcelains are applied to the gold coloured coping. As with the Golden Gate System and Sunrise Crown there is some reflection from the gold coping, which can enhance aesthetics. Unlike conventional cast metal ceramic restorations, tooth preparation can be reduced significantly, it being possible to make crown margins 0.3 mm wide. However,

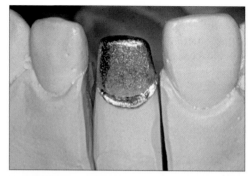

Fig. 5 A Captek coping for a ceramo-metal restoration of a central incisor. The buccal margin will be thinned to a micro-margin prior to porcelain application. Captek is unusual in that it resists firing distortion resulting from differential thermal contraction of metal and porcelain.

our experience with the material shows that it can be difficult to obtain a good crown margin unless an obvious chamfer or shoulder is present.

The manufacturer's literature quotes a study from the University of Boston, which compares restorations, made from Captek with those made from a high quality palladium-containing alloy. The sheer bond strength of porcelain to Captek was almost twice as high whilst crowns of both materials loaded at the incisal edge showed similar load bearing characteristics. Marginal fit was also reported to be excellent and significantly better than conventional

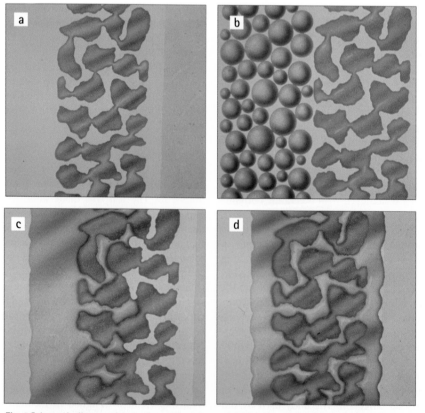

Fig. 6 Schematic diagram showing how a Captek core is laid down as gold alloy impregnated wax sheets: a) the granular appearance of Captek W after the first wax layer has been burnt off; b) application of the second wax layer (Captek G); c) perfusion of the Captek W by the Captek G during the second firing; and d) the resulting composite metal structure after firing (Courtesy of Schottlander).

metal ceramic crowns. Long-term studies are needed to confirm anecdotal evidence of good clinical performance. Occlusal contacts are usually formed in ceramic, as metal contacts are difficult to build.

Electroformed copings
The GES Gold Electroforming System uses an ionic solution to electroplate a 0.3mm thickness of pure gold directly onto the die. The die is coated with a metallic silver varnish to render it conductive. The manufacturers claim a similar strength characteristic to type III gold but the system is not supported by any clinical studies.

Strengthening of feldspathic metal-ceramic porcelains
Feldspathic porcelains are inherently weak in tension and strong in compression. Hence they rely on bonding to metal and coping design to dissipate tensile stresses. Another approach is to generate compressive stresses either internally or in the immediate subsurface layer. A recent innovation is the use of ion exchange where smaller diameter sodium ions in the surface of the porcelain are replaced by larger diameter potassium ions. This exchange has the potential to strengthen by subsurface compression, however any strengthening effect is lost if the restoration is subsequently self-glazed or finished. Surprisingly, the ion exchange technique does not give a significantly greater increase in flexural strength than simple overglazing.[76] Where overglazing is not practical, fine polishing with diamond pastes helps remove surface flaws and gives a modest increase in strength over self-glazing.

RESIN COMPOSITES
The use of resin composites for indirect inlays and onlays is well known.[77] Recently, manufacturers have introduced highly filled composite materials for making indirect crowns and bridges. Clearly the major advantage is in reduced laboratory costs, but it should also be born in mind that modern composites induce much less wear against opposing teeth than porcelain. It is too early to say whether these materials will perform well in the long-term, however they at very least offer a good solution where restorations are not expected to last for extended periods eg young patients. Materials falling into this category include Artglass, and Targis and Vectris. The Vectis material is interesting in that it uses a silanated glass fibre mat reinforcement for crowns and glass fibre strands to give strength to bridge spans.

Finally, several systems have been developed for bonding composite to metal substructures. These include the Silicoater and Kevloc techniques which both require specialised laboratory equipment. Restorations of this type are more popular in continental Europe than in the UK where metal-ceramics predominate.

CONCLUSION
With more and more materials being introduced it is important that dentists understand the variety available and the factors which will contribute to the success or failure of their restorations. In the final analysis established or promising materials should be subjected to randomised clinical trial. Several manufacturers are adopting this approach but more need to do so. While there is considerable clinical research data on intra-coronal restorations much more is needed on those placed extra-coronally.

1. O'Brien W. Evolution of dental casting. In: Valega T, editor. *Alternatives to gold alloys in dentistry,* Conf. Proc. DHEW Pub. No. [NIH]77-1227. Washington DC: U.S. Government Printing Office, 1977.
2. Craig G, O'Brien W, Powers J. *Dental Materials properties and manipulation.* pp.236-250. St Louis: Mosby, 1983.
3. Cohen S, Kakar A, Vaidyanathan T, Viswanadhan T. Castability optimization of palladium based alloys. *J Prosthet Dent* 1996; **76:** 125-131.
4. Marzouk M, Saleh L, Emanuel R, Malone W. Clinical behaviour of silver-palladium alloy castings: a five year comparative clinical study. J Prosthet Dent 1991; **65:** 19-26.
5. Kansu G, Aydin A. Evaluation of the biocompatibility of various dental alloys: part II - allergenic potentials. *Eur J Prosthodont Rest Dent* 1996; **4:** 155-161.
6. Mulders C, Darwish M, Holze R. Corrosion behaviour of dental alloys - an in-vitro study. *J Oral Rehabil* 1996; **23:** 825-831.
7. Frykholm K, Frithiof L, Fernström A, Moberger G, Blohm S, Björn E. Allergy to copper derived from dental alloys as a possible cause of oral lesions of lichen planus. *Acta Dermato-Venereologica* 1969; **49:** 268-281.
8. Smart E, Macleod R, Lawrence C. Resolution of lichen planus following removal of amalgam restorations in patients with proven allergy to mercury salts: a pilot study. *Br Dent J* 1995; **178:** 108-112.
9. Pierce L, Goodkind R. A status report of the possible risks of base metal alloys and their components. *J Prosthet Dent* 1989; **62:** 234-237.
10. Northeast S E, van Noort R, Johnson A, Winstanley R B, White GE. Metal-ceramic bridges from commercial dental laboratories: alloy composition, cost and quality of fit. *Br Dent J* 1992; **172:** 198-204.
11. Nery S, McCabe J F, Wassell R W. A comparative study of three dental adhesives. *J Dent* 1994; **23:** 55-61.
12. Weiss P. New design parameters: utilising the properties of Ni-Cr super alloys. *Dent Clin N Am* 1977; **21:** 749.
13. Kelly J, Rose T. Nonprecious alloys for use in fixed prosthodontics: a literature review. *J Prosthet Dent* 1983; **49:** 363-370.
14. Equipment. CoDMIa. Report on base metal alloys for crown and bridge applications: benefits and risks. *J Am Dent Assoc* 1985; **111:** 479-483.
15. Wiltshire W, Ferriera M, Ligthelm A J. Allergies to dental materials. *Quintessence Int* 1996; **27:** 513-520.
16. Ida K, Togaya T, Tsutsumi S, Takeuchi M. Effect of magnesia investments in the dental casting of pure titanium or titanium alloys. *Dent Mater J* 1982; **1:** 8-21.
17. Ida K, Tani Y, Tsutsumi S. Clinical application of pure Ti-crowns. *Dent Mater J* 1985; **4:** 191-195.
18. Andersson M, Bergman B, Bessing C, Ericson G, Lundquist P, Nilson H. Clinical results with titanium crowns fabricated with machine duplication and spark erosion. *Acta Odontol Scand* 1989; **47:** 279-286.
19. Bergman B, Bessing C, Ericson G, Lundquist P, Nilson H, Andersson M. A two year follow up study of titanium crowns. *Acta Odontol Scand* 1990; **48:** 113-117.
20. Michalske T, Freiman S. A molecular interpretation of stress corrosion in silica. *Nature* 1982; **295:** 511-512.
21. McClean J, Hughes T. The reinforcement of dental porcelain with ceramic oxides. *Br Dent J* 1965; **119:** 251-267.
22. Denry I. Recent advances in ceramics for dentistry. *Crit Rev Oral Biol Med* 1996; **7:** 134-143.
23. Jones D, Wilson H J. Some properties of dental ceramics. *J Oral Rehabil* 1975; **2:** 379-396.
24. Anusavice K, Zang N, Moorhead J. Influence of colorants on crystallization and mechanical properties of lithia-based glass ceramics. *Dent Mater* 1994; **10:** 141-146.
25. Denry I, Rosensteil S. Flexural strength and fracture

RESIN COMPOSITES
KEY POINT:
• Improvements in technology (including fibre filler) look promising but require long-term evaluation

toughness of Dicor glass-ceramic after embedment modification. *J Dent Res* 1993; **72:** 572-576.

26. Geller W K, Kwiatkowski S J. The Willi's glass crown: a new solution in the dark and shadowed zone of aesthetic porcelain restorations. *Quintessence Dent Tech* 1987; **11:** 233-242.

27. Al-Shehri S, Mohammed H, Wilson C. Influence of lamination on the flexural strength of a dental castable glass-ceramic. *J Prosthet Dent* 1996; **76:** 23-28.

28. Dong J, Luthy H, Wohlwend A, Sharer P. Heat-pressed ceramics: technology and strength. *Int J Prosthodont* 1992; **5:** 9-16.

29. Qualtrough A, Piddock V. Dental CAD/CAM: A millstone or a milestone? *Dent Update* 1995; **22:** 200-204.

30. Mormann W, Krejci K. Computer designed inlays after 5 years in situ: clinical performance and scanning electron microscopic evaluation. *Quintessence Int* 1992; **23:** 109-115.

31. Sjögren S, Bergman M, Molin M, Bessing C A. A clinical examination of ceramic (Cerac) Inlays. *Acta Odontol Scand* 1992; **50:** 171-178.

32. Isenberg B P, Essig M E, Leinfelder K F. Three year clinical evaluation of CAD/CAM restorations. *J Aesthet Dent* 1992; **4:** 173-176.

33. Inokoshi S, B. VM, Willems G, Lambrechts P, Braem M, Vanherles G. Marginal accuracy of CAD/CAM inlays made with the original and the updated software. *J Dent* 1992; **20:** 171-177.

34. Thompson J, Bayne S, Heymann H. Mechanical properties of new mica-based machinable glass ceramic of CAD/CAM restorations. *J Prosthet Dent* 1996; **76:** 619-623.

35. Tinschert J, Zwez D, Marx R, Anusavice K J. Structural reliability of alumina-, feldspar-, leucite-, mica- and zirconia-based ceramics. *J Dent* 2000; **28:** 529-535.

36. Wagner W, Chu T. Biaxial flexural strength and indentation toughness of three new dental core ceramics. *J Prosthet Dent* 1996; **76:** 140-141.

37. Brunton P A, Smith P, McCord J F, Wilson N H F. Procera all-ceramic crowns: a new approach to an old problem. *Br Dent J* 1999; **186:** 430-434.

38. ISO. International standard 6872-1984. *Dental Ceramic.* 1st ed. pp.1-14. Geneva, Switzerland: International Organisation for Standardization, 1984.

39. Ban S, Anusavice K J. Influence of test method on failure stress of brittle dental materials. *J Dent Res* 1990; **69:** 1791-1799.

40. McClean J, Jeansonne E, Chiche G, Pinault A. All ceramic crowns and foil crowns. *In:* Chiche G, Pinault A, editors. *Esthetics of anterior fixed prosthodontics.* pp.97-113. Chicago: Quintessence Publishing Co., Inc., 1994.

41. Brandson S J, King P A. The impact fracture resistance of restored endodontically treated anterior teeth. *J Dent Res* 1992; **72:** 1141.

42. Madani M, Chu F C, McDonald A V, Smales R J. Effects of surface treatments on shear bond strengths between a resin cement and an alumina core. *J Prosthet Dent* 2000; **83:** 644-647.

43. Blixt M, Adamczak E, Linden L A, Oden A, Arvidson K. Bonding to densely sintered alumina surfaces: effect of sandblasting and silica coating on shear bond strength of luting cements. *Int J Prosthodont* 2000; **13:** 221-226.

44. Karlsson S. The fit of Procera titanium crowns. *Acta Odontol Scand* 1993; **51:** 129-134.

45. McClean J W, von Fraunhofer J A. The estimation of cement film thickness by an in vivo technique. *Br Dent J* 1971; **131:** 107-111.

46. Christensen G J. Marginal fit of gold inlay castings. *J Prosthet Dent* 1966; **16:** 297-305.

47. White S N, Kipnis V. Influence of marginal opening on microleakage of cemented artificial crowns. *J Prosthet Dent* 1994; **71:** 257-264.

48. Björn AL, Björn H, Grkovik B. Marginal fit of restorations and its relation to periodontal bone level. *Odont Rev* 1970; **21:** 337-346.

49. 147/242. PoCN, Morris H F. Department of Veterans Affairs Cooperative Studies Project No. 242. Quantitative and qualitative evaluation of cast ceramic, porcelain-shoulder, and cast metal full crown margins. *J Prosthet Dent* 1992; **67:** 198-203.

50. Holmes R J, Sulik W D, Holland G A, Bayne S C. Marginal fit of castable ceramic crowns. *J Prosthet Dent* 1992; **67:** 594-599.

51. Castellani D, Baccetti T, Clauser C, Bernadini U D. Thermal distortion of different materials in crown construction. *J Prosthet Dent* 1994; **72:** 360-366.

52. Shearer B, Gough M B, Setchell D J. Influence of marginal configuration and porcelain addition on the fit of In-Ceram crowns. *Biomater* 1996; **17:** 1891-1895.

53. Ratledge D, Smith B, Wilson R. The effect of restorative materials on the wear of human enamel. *J Prosthet Dent* 1994; **72:** 194-203.

54. Monasky G, Taylor D. Studies on the wear of porcelain, enamel and gold. *J Prosthet Dent* 1971; **25:** 299-306.

55. Seghi R, Rosensteil S, Bauer P. Abrasion of human enamel by different dental ceramics in vitro. *J Dent Res* 1991; **70:** 221-225.

56. Krejci I, Lutz F, Reimer M. Wear of CAD/CAM ceramic inlays: restorations, opposing cusps and luting cements. *Quintessence Int* 1994; **25:** 199-207.

57. Hacker C H, Wagner W C, Razoog M E. An *in-vitro* investigation of the wear of enamel on porcelain and gold in saliva. *J Prosthet Dent* 1996; **75:** 14-17.

58. Al-Hiyasatt A S. *An investigation of the wear of human enamel and dental ceramics.* [PhD]. University of Glasgow, 1997.

59. Probster L. Four year clinical study of glass infiltrated, sintered alumina crowns. *J Oral Rehabil* 1996; **23:** 147-151.

60. McLaren E A, White S N. Survival of In-Ceram crowns in a private practice: a prospective clinical trial. *J Prosthet Dent* 2000; **83:** 216-22.

61. Oden A, Andersson M, Krystek-Ondracek I, Magnusson D. Five-year clinical evaluation of Procera AllCeram crowns. *J Prosthet Dent* 1998; **80:** 450-6.

62. Brecker S C. Porcelain baked to gold: a new medium in prosthodontics. *J Prosthet Dent* 1956; **6:** 801-810.

63. Weinstein M, Weinstein A. Ney Company, assignee. Fused Porcelain-to-metal teeth. US Patent 3,052,982, September 11. 1962.

64. Pang I, Gilbert J, Chai J, Lautenschlager E. Bonding characteristics of low-fusing porcelain bonded to pure titanium and palladium-copper alloy. *J Prosthet Dent* 1995; **73:** 17-25.

65. Walter M, Reppel P D, Boning K, Freesmeyer W B. Six-year follow-up of titanium and high-gold porcelain-fused-to-metal fixed partial dentures. *J Oral Rehabil* 1999; **26:** 91-96.

66. Mattmuller A, Wassmann J, Biffar R. Hydrothermal ceramic for porcelain-fused- to-metal crowns: an initial experience report from clinical practice. *Quintessence Int* 1996; **27:** 521-526.

67. McClean J, Sced I. The bonded alumina crown. 1. The bonding of platinum to aluminous dental porcelain using tin oxide coatings. *Aust Dent J* 1976; **21:** 119-127.

68. McClean J, Kedge M, Hubbard J. The bonded alumina crown. 2. Construction using the twin foil technique. *Aust Dent J* 1976; **21:** 262-263.

69. Philp G, Brukl C. Compressive strengths of conventional, twin foil, and all-ceramic crowns. *J Prosthet Dent* 1984; **52:** 215-220.

70. Piddock V, Marquis P, Wilson H. Comparison of the strengths of aluminous porcelain fired onto platinum and palladium foils. *J Oral Rehabil* 1991; **13:** 31-37.

71. Southan D. Defects in porcelain at the porcelain-to-metal interface. *In:* Yamada H, Grenoble P, editors. *Dental porcelain: the state of the art - 1977.* pp.48-49. Los Angeles: University of Southern California, 1977.

72. Hopkins K. A method of strengthening aluminous porcelain jacket crowns. *Br Dent J* 1981; **151:** 225-227.

73. Hummert T, Barghi N, Berry T. Effect of fitting adjustments on compressive strength of a new foil crown system. *J Prosthet Dent* 1991; **66:** 177-180.

74. Hummert T, Barghi N, Berry T. Postcementation marginal fit of a new ceramic foil crown system. *J Prosthet Dent* 1992; **68:** 766-770.

75. Shoher I, Whiteman A. Captek - A new capillary casting technology for ceramometal restorations. *Quintessence Dent Tech* 1995; **18:** 9-20.

76. Giordano R A, Campbell S, Pober R. Flexural strength of feldspathic porcelain treated with ion exchange, overglaze, and polishing. *J Prosthet Dent* 1994; **71:** 468-472.

77. Burke F, Watts D, Wilson N, Wilson M. Current status and rationale for composite inlays and onlays. *Br Dent J* 1991; **170:** 269-273.

78. EH40/97. *Occupational exposure limits 1997 for use with The Control of Substances Hazardous to Health Regulations 1994.* pp.14-17. Sudbury: HSE Books, 1997.

79. Seghi R, Daher T, Caputo A. Relative flexural strength of dental restorative ceramics. *Dent Mater* 1990; **6:** 181-184.

80. Seghi R, Sorensen J. Relative flexural strength of six new ceramic materials. *Int J Prosthodont* 1995; **8:** 239-246.

81. Wohlwend A, Strub J, Scharer P. Metal ceramic and all porcelain restorations: current considerations. *Int J Prosthodont* 1989; **2:** 13-26.

List of products mentioned in the text

Alceram	Innotek Dental Corp., Lakewood, USA
Artglass	Heraeus Kulzer, Wehrheim, Germany
Captek	Schottlander, Letchworth, UK
Cerapearl	Kyocera, San Diego, USA
Corning MGC-F	Corning Inc., New York, USA
Dicor	Corning Inc., New York, USA
Dicor MGC	Corning Inc., New York, USA
Dicor Plus	Corning Inc., New York, USA
Duceratin	Degussa AG, Frankfurt, Germany
Duceram-LFC	Degussa AG, Frankfurt, Germany
Duceragold	Degussa AG, Frankfurt, Germany
GES Gold	Gramm Technology, 75233 Tiefenbronn, Germany
Hi-Ceram	Vita Zahnfabrik, D-79704 Bad Säckingen, Germany
In-Ceram	Vita Zahnfabrik, D-79704 Bad Säckingen, Germany
In-Ceram Spinnel	Vita Zahnfabrik, D-79704 Bad Säckingen, Germany
In-Ceram Zirconia	Vita Zahnfabrik, D-79704 Bad Säckingen, Germany
IPS Empress	Ivoclar-Vivadent, Schaan, Liechtenstein
Kevlock	Heraeus Kulzer GmbH, Wehrheim/Ts, Germany
Mirage II	Myron International, Kansas City, USA
Optec HSP	Jeneric/Pentron Inc., Wallingford, USA
Procera AllCeram	Nobel Biocare, Göteburg, Sweden
Procera Porcelain	Nobel Biocare, Göteburg, Sweden
Silicoater	Heraeus Kulzer GmbH, Wehrheim/Ts, Germany
Sunrise Foil Crown	Tanaka Dental Products, Skokie, USA
Targis/Vectris	Ivoclar-Vivadent, Schaan, Liechtenstein
Techceram	Techceram Ltd., Shipley, UK
Vitadur-N	Vita Zahnfabrik, D-79704 Bad Säckingen, Germany
Vita Mark II	Vita Zahnfabrik, D-79704 Bad Säckingen, Germany

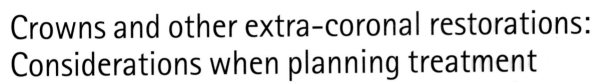

IN BRIEF

- A long-term view of crown provision is essential (ten years or more)
- Meeting the patient's expectations is a critical measure of success
- The patient's ability to tolerate treatment and maintain the restorations is a key factor when planning treatment
- One's own ability to provide high quality crowns requires honest reflection in every case
- The damage to tooth tissue when providing crowns is considerable and should be weighed against the benefits
- Control of the environment to minimise disease and damage is a fundamental part of the treatment plan
- The biological and biomechanical safety of the restorations is taken as a prerequisite

Crowns and other extra-coronal restorations: Considerations when planning treatment

D. J. Jacobs[1] J. G. Steele[2] and R. W. Wassell[3]

Considerations when planning treatment is the third in the series of crowns and other extra-coronal restorations. Articles or chapters on treatment planning in restorative dentistry can make pretty dry reading, often built around a list of factors that might influence your decision-making. In truth though, planning and placing crowns or other extra-coronal restorations cannot be distilled into a series of lists. The decision-making involved requires experience, subtle understanding and a flexible approach, none of which come easily.

[1]*Consultant in Restorative Dentistry, Newcastle Dental Hospital, Richardson Road, Newcastle upon Tyne NE2 4AZ
[2]Senior Lecturer in Restorative Dentistry,
[3]Senior Lecturer in Restorative Dentistry, Department of Restorative Dentistry, The Dental School, Framlington Place, Newcastle upon Tyne NE2 4BW
*Correspondence to: D. J. Jacobs
E-mail: D.J.Jacobs@ncl.ac.uk

No crowns can really be regarded as permanent. If we lived for long enough, wear and tear, disease and the realities of intra-oral existence mean that even the most carefully constructed and cemented crown would probably eventually fail. We should though expect to get many useful years from our crowns, and should plan to have a situation we can recover, if and when they eventually fail. This article aims to address the issues of planning, both by planning to avoid failure and also by planning to cope with failure. It will address both the treatment plan itself and the planned delivery of treatment (these are subtly different things), and it aims to set the scene for the more detailed and specific analysis of treatment planning and delivery issues within the rest of this series of articles.

Learning is most effective when you learn from your mistakes, but this can be a painful process, both for patient and operator. Here we will use examples where mistakes have been made (some quite close to home) to illustrate the points we are trying to make. Take a few moments to look at the illustrations of the two cases shown, and read the text in the boxes.

Many of the cases that fail miserably suffer from decisions made right at the beginning. In other cases the decisions are sound but the execution is the problem. These two cases were abject failures at several points and illustrate, perhaps in a rather extreme way, some of the fundamentals of planning. One was done in a dental hospital, the other in a practice. Bad planning and bad execution were contributors in both. We will refer to these two cases as we go through.

THE LONG-TERM STRATEGY: WHAT WILL THIS DENTITION BE LIKE IN 10 YEARS?

A long-term strategy is different from a treatment plan. It is temptingly easy to focus immediately at the level of the tooth, discussing its crown height, pulp vitality or its role in the occlusion. Whilst these detailed 'close focus' issues are all critically important if a crown is to survive, they are not as important as making a decision about treating the tooth in the context of the rest of the dentition, and about managing the rest of the dentition in the context of the individual.

Look at Case 1 (see box overleaf). This failed for many reasons, including poor technical outcomes and perhaps insufficient attention to hygiene and diet. But as you look at the first radiograph, ask yourself this question: 'if this patient attended my surgery now, what condition would I expect this dentition to be in, in 10 years time?' The answer might be 'edentulous', it may be that there will be a couple of remaining teeth and an overdenture, but the answer probably is not 'the same as it is now'. Given the widespread caries and the lack of remaining sound tooth tissue, tooth loss here was always very likely. Had this been acknowledged right at the beginning, rather than trying to save and re-crown every tooth (and on a 'close focus' tooth-by-tooth basis this seemed quite possible no doubt), then a reasonable end stage would have been reached more quickly, more efficiently and less traumatically. Who knows, implants may not have been necessary if the transition to edentulousness had been planned, or a couple of overdenture abutments had been identified at the start. If you ask yourself: 'What

A guide to crowns

CASE 1

In 1989 this patient had all of her lower teeth crowned.

Two years later there was evidence of caries around the margins of several of them (Fig. 1).

A further decision was made to root treat all of the teeth, initially with a view to restoring them with crowns and this treatment was started a short time later, initially leaving the crowns in place (Fig. 2).

The root treatments were undertaken, but within a year they began to fail because, among many other reasons, it was proving very difficult to ensure a coronal seal (Fig. 3), in fact it is doubtful whether this biological pre-requisite to successful endodontics had been considered at all.

As no progress was being made (things were actually getting worse), the decision was made to revert to an overdenture (Fig. 4).

Within another year even the overdenture abutments became mobile and infected (Fig. 5) and in the end they too were removed, leaving the patient with a denture which she could not wear.

The end result, a further 2 years down the line, was the placement of four implants and a very successful lower implant retained fixed prosthesis (Fig. 6).

The whole case cost several thousand pounds to manage, much of which was used to provide treatment which soon failed.

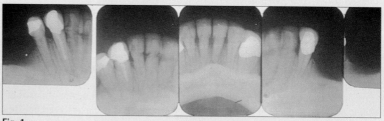
Fig. 1

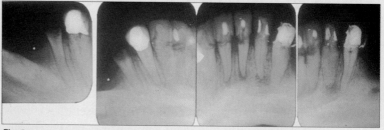
Fig. 2

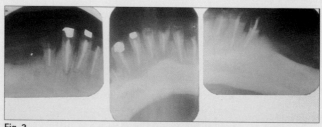
Fig. 3

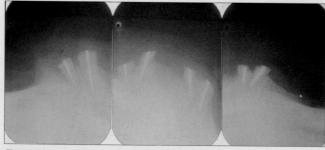
Fig. 4

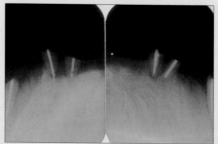
Fig. 5

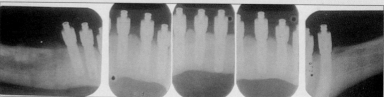
Fig. 6

will this be like in 10 years, or 20?' and can answer, a sensible strategy for how you want to get there can be developed.

Essentially this is gambling, a game of odds. You cannot possibly hope to know what things will be like in 10 years, can you? Perhaps not, but as a professional you are better placed to assess the 'form' of the dentition than anyone else. Often, it is unwise to develop your final strategy straight away, before you have seen the response to basic preventive measures such as hygiene and dietary management. Increasingly we find that the 'one off' treatment plan is actually inappropriate, as it was in the case in Figure 7 where isolated coronal restorations and bridgework have been provided in an environment of generalised toothwear. This clearly warranted fuller investigation and an overall management strategy. Taking your time and planning in stages, will often improve your chances of winning this game of odds.

With a strategy in place, it is now time to ask some more specific questions, starting with some issues relating to the patient as a whole before finally moving on to technicalities associated with the patient's mouth and teeth.

CASE SELECTION: THE PATIENT

Can I meet the expectations of the patient?
The first fundamental issue that you need to resolve with the patient is whether your expectations and theirs converge. It is all very well being able to sell something to your patient, but you have to be able to deliver and, in the long term, 'expectation modification' can be a key skill. The issue of expectations most often arises in terms of aesthetics (see Part 6 in this series) though there are issues in other areas too. We know that patients' expectations for tooth retention are increasing all the time,[1] and this applies as much to treatment decisions on individual teeth as it does to the dentition as a whole. Where you really feel that expectations cannot be met or modified it is better to make an appropriate referral at the beginning than risk later retribution.

Will the patient be able to tolerate the treatment and then maintain the restorations?
Planning some restorations based on the technicalities of pulp state, angulation, crown height and so on is all very well, but if the patient cannot lie flat for more than 20 minutes, or cannot open their mouth beyond 2 centimetres, actually providing treatment may cause you some problems. It is surprisingly easy to forget to think these things through before lifting a handpiece. Physical limitations, such as neuromuscular or skeletal disorders, may also prevent patients from maintaining their restorations, no matter how devoted they are to good hygiene. Furthermore, it is not simply the state of hygiene you encounter when you see the patient for the first time that matters, it is also how you see them being able to cope in 5 or 10 years. This may not be an issue for young or middle-aged patients,

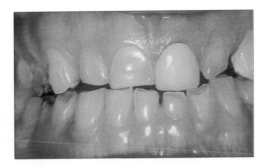

Fig. 7 'isolated coronal restorations and bridgework with generalised toothwear'

but for an increasingly dentate and demanding group of older adults it is highly relevant. The treatment planning strategy of 'shortened dental arch' (SDA) is built around the differences in the ease with which different types of tooth can be maintained and cleaned. Anterior teeth are easier for the dentist to access for treatment and long-term maintenance and for the patient to clean. Molars on the other hand are difficult. They have multiple roots with furcations between them, as well as fine and curved root canals. Their inaccessible location means that, if there are real problems cleaning, these are the teeth most likely to suffer. SDA gives priority to the anterior and premolar teeth to ensure that limited resources are targeted to the teeth which have the best chance of long-term survival, and which will provide adequate mechanical and aesthetic function.

My own skills: Can I do this to a high enough standard?
This can be a difficult question to face up to but it is a question that should be answered honestly. Tackling a complex case requiring multiple coronal restorations with an excess of bravado and a lack of insight and understanding of the potential pitfalls can lead to disaster. Good restorative work is more than being able to cut some shapes and stick on crowns. Dentistry is difficult. The knowledge and experience, not to mention the technical skills that are required to make the complex judgements necessary to plan and then carry out treatment take a long time to acquire. Other factors, which enter the equation and may affect the outcome, include the availability of adequate treatment facilities, materials and appropriate technical support. Ultimately the decision is yours, but there is usually more than one treatment option and simpler alternatives may be more successful in the long-term.

Can I justify the damage I am going to do to the patient's teeth?
Look at Case 2 again (see box overleaf). This is a case where a decision was made to place crowns on perfectly sound teeth. Admittedly, the clinical work was poor, but the resultant damage was almost terminal for the teeth. This was a planning failure every bit as much as a clinical failure. It is easy to be seduced by the technical possibilities and to forget the biological realities when creating a treatment plan. In a recent review of patients visiting a UK dental hospital, 19% of all crowned teeth without root fillings had evidence of periapical

CASE 2

This 18-year-old female patient attended Newcastle Dental Hospital requesting treatment to improve the appearance of her upper anterior teeth which were chipped as a result of trauma with UL1 (21) having been root filled and discoloured (Fig. 8). She was placed on a waiting list for conservative management involving the provision of a labial porcelain veneer to UL1 (21) and incisal composite restorations to UR1 (11), UR2 (12) and UL2 (22).

Inevitable delays with treatment at the Dental Hospital led to the patient seeking treatment elsewhere. She did, however, return to the Dental Hospital some 5 years later with PJCs of poor quality on all the upper anterior teeth and irreversible pulpitis in UR2 (12) and UL2 (22) (Fig. 9). A further treatment plan was formulated involving endodontics to UR2 (12) and UL2 (22) followed by replacement crowns for the upper anterior teeth. Once again, Dental Hospital waiting lists resulted in the patient obtaining treatment elsewhere. A further 8 years later, she was referred back to the Dental Hospital by her latest dentist who was suitably horrified by what he found! The results of 13 years of treatment were six poor crowns with carious margins, unrootfilled or inadequately rootfilled teeth, short or perforating posts and several teeth of very doubtful prognosis (Fig. 10). In summary, an unnecessarily mutilated dentition.

Fortunately, remedial treatment from her own dentist was possible in this case and the result is much better than could have been hoped for initially (Fig. 11). This is also a very good illustration of what can be achieved in the General Dental Services under ideal circumstances although it is important to note that the treatment required a further 17 visits over a 9-month period, including two surgical procedures, and the longevity of the restorations remains unpredictable.

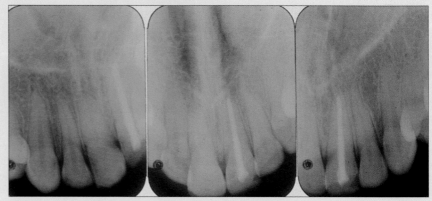

Fig. 8

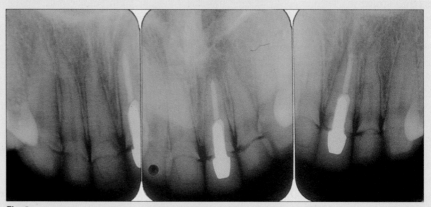

Fig. 9

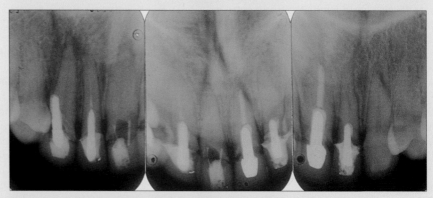

Fig. 10

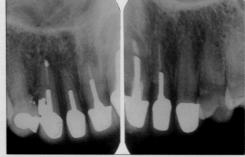

Fig. 11

pathology.[2] For a number of technical reasons it is very difficult to get an accurate indication of just how often teeth die as a result of crown preparation, but this finding and other published evidence suggests it is probably a fairly common occurrence, unless the technical quality of the work is of a very high standard.[3,4] Furthermore, the tooth itself is often weakened by preparation, and fracture of the tooth at gum level is not uncommon. Crown preparation on virgin teeth is not something to be undertaken lightly.

What is the main lesson to be learnt from Case 2? We have already stated in the introduction that all crowns may eventually fail but the poor standard of clinical work in this instance has certainly resulted in unacceptable early and damaging failure. The message is clear that if there are simpler, less invasive, but effective means of achieving the desired result, as there were in this case, these should always be considered before embarking upon more complex treatments which may actually accelerate the loss of the dentition.

CASE SELECTION: THE MOUTH AND TEETH

The oral environment: Can I, and the patient, control the environment to minimise the risk of disease or damage in the long term?

It is tempting sometimes to want to crack on and do the difficult, skilled and lucrative technical things, to see the final result, and to witness the transformed smile. The new crowns though are only as good as their environment. Sometimes it takes a lot of time to sort out the environment, for little immediate reward. At other times you just have to work within a difficult environment; for example it may be rather difficult to stop a bruxist from grinding and you may need to plan around this. Usually you have to accept less than perfection, often much less, but plaque control, caries risk and the occlusion are at the heart of successful crown work. All can be managed to some degree. If you should be in any doubt about the importance of managing the environment, look again at Case 1 where neither plaque control, nor caries management were properly dealt with. The result was time consuming and expensive failure.

Is the plaque control good enough?
Little needs to be said about plaque. We know that it is a fundamental factor in both caries and periodontal disease. In simple terms, plaque around restorations is likely to shorten their life. Tooth cleaning is a surprisingly complex process, and sometimes we forget this or even trivialise it. Helping people to find the skills to keep their own teeth clean is probably the least trivial thing dentists do.

It is truly remarkable that any form of operative dentistry should be considered in an environment like this (Fig. 12), let alone the provision of crowns that have been carefully contoured to follow the aberrant gingival margins! The pres-

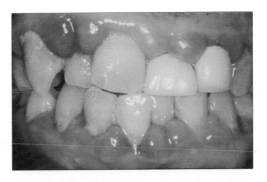

Fig. 12 'poor oral hygiene and crowns'

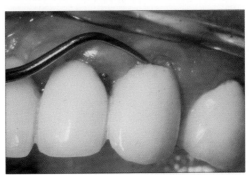

Fig. 13 'deficient margins and recurrent caries'

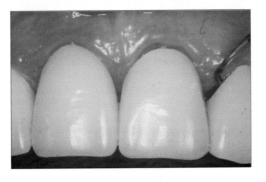

Fig. 14 'deficient margins with good plaque control'

ence of marginal deficiencies in an environment where plaque control is inadequate can result in rapid caries progression and potential tooth loss (Fig. 13). Contrast this situation with Figure 14 which illustrates poor open crown margins but where caries is minimal. Again, this quality of treatment cannot be condoned but the saving grace has been the patient's maintenance of a high standard of plaque control.

It is the dentist's responsibility to provide the highest standard of technical work possible, but also to communicate to the patient the importance of good hygiene and maintenance. The patient's responsibility is to follow that advice on the understanding that they may directly influence the longevity of their dental restorations. The fact that they may have made a considerable investment in terms of time and expense for their dental treatment represents a powerful incentive to comply with future preventive measures.

Has the risk of caries in the future been addressed?
Caries risk is directly related to both plaque and diet, and also (in the case of root caries) to the presence of a partial denture.[5-7] The oral health profile of most western populations is such that our crown patients of the next few decades will,

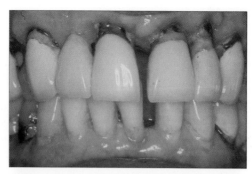

Fig. 15 'root caries and attempted repairs'

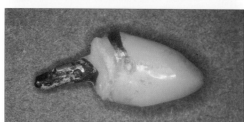

Fig. 16 'de-bonded anterior post crown'

for the most part, be a steadily ageing band.[1] Caries management is an issue at all ages, but in this cohort root caries is likely to be an increasing threat. This is a wretched disease to deal with. The best crown in the world, with an undetectable margin, perfect occlusion and stunning aesthetics will still fail if the risk of root caries is not addressed. In this case (Fig. 15), the risk of caries around the upper anterior restorations has clearly not been properly addressed with root caries and progressive periodontal destruction resulting. Treatment has involved the mechanical repair of caries at the crown margins (and in some areas the repair of the repairs) with little or no emphasis on prevention. The solution for managing root caries is biological not mechanical. It requires simple communication about hygiene and attention to some 'little things' in the diet, such as the odd teaspoon of sugar in regular cups of tea or coffee, biscuit nibbling and a range of other apparently innocuous activities which patients may not associate with a problem. If you are in any doubt as to how important this is, just scan Case 1 again. The dentist has at his or her disposal a full armamentarium of approaches, including hygiene and dietary advice and the appropriate use of fluorides and varnishes. Caries, particularly root caries, is preventable. If your crowns fail because of caries it is partly a failure of your own management.

Has the risk of damage from the occlusion been minimised?
A few basic checks and a little thought and care should eliminate the risk of problems in the large majority of cases. It is important that you know where the contacts are on the tooth you are to treat, especially those that are involved in guiding the jaw movement in lateral and protrusive excursions. It is also important to know which other teeth are involved in guidance, and whether the tooth you are about to prepare is a deflective contact or interference to guidance. These may sound complex but are readily checked and there is rarely a problem. Tech-

niques for occlusal examination and adjustment are dealt with in Part 5.

Figure 16 shows a de-bonded anterior post crown. Many kilos of zinc phosphate must be used and many unnecessary hours spent re-cementing such restorations. Often the blame is put on a short or non-retentive post (which this tooth shows), but in our experience a large proportion dislodge because inadequate care is taken to ensure that it is not providing all of the anterior guidance. Look at the profile of the palatal surface of this crown, it is bulky and convex and it is difficult to believe that this complied with the natural pattern of guidance provided by the adjacent natural teeth. Although the post is not long, the contour of the guidance surface must have been a contributory factor. Any anterior tooth is likely to provide some element of protrusive guidance and you can and should spend a few moments thinking about how to manage this right at the outset. Again details are given in Part 5.

The nature of the opposing tooth contacts is also important in terms of the material used for the occlusal/palatal surfaces of coronal restorations. In this case (Figs 17,18) there is already an ongoing toothwear problem caused by erosion and the provision of upper anterior crowns with porcelain palatal surfaces, which have been adjusted to make them even more abrasive, is not a good example of planning and the potential for further wear is self-evident.

The tooth: Are the foundations biologically and biomechanically sound?
The periodontal tissues
A tooth with any amount of attachment loss can be crowned, but where the disease is advanced and uncontrolled it is a hopeless investment. The major issues though do not surround the risk to

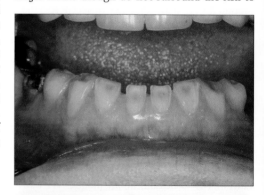

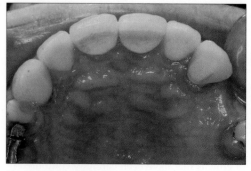

Figure 17,18 'worn dentition with porcelain abrasion'

your crown from periodontal disease but the risk to the periodontal tissues from your crown. Poor crown margins can certainly result in gingival problems (Fig. 19), as can an incorrect emergence profile. All crown margins should, ideally, be placed supragingivally to avoid problems related to gingival inflammation. Where a subgingival margin is indicated, it is essential that the margin be placed within the limits of the sulcus and that the biologic width is not encroached upon (Fig. 20). The biologic width is a band of approximately 2 mm of supracrestal connective tissue attachment and junctional epithelium around every tooth. If a restoration encroaches upon or eliminates this 2 mm band of attachment, an inflammatory response occurs and attachment loss, apical migration and pocket formation may result. Contrast the healthy gingivae associated with the supragingival crown margin on tooth UR1 (11) in Fig. 21 with the subgingival margin on tooth UL1 (21). Marginal position is something to be planned in advance, and as a rule of thumb it is wise to minimise encroachment into the sulcus.

Apart from encouraging periodontal problems, the subgingival placement of margins can also make accurate impression recording difficult or impossible. In Figure 22 subgingival margin placement has led to gingival inflammation, either as a result of biologic width encroachment or poor marginal fit resulting from obvious difficulties with impressions, as in Figure 23. Poorly contoured temporaries can also result in problems with impressions because of poor gingival condition (Fig. 24). The replacement of such restorations with well fitting and contoured provisional restorations may need to be a planned first step prior to definitive treatment.

Is the endodontic state stable enough to allow a crown to be planned?
Managing the endodontic state can be a particularly difficult problem, in fact we have devoted an entire article to the subject (see Part 4). Generally speaking though, for vital teeth the issues are quite straightforward. The pulp is a living tissue and everyone's life is easier where it remains a living tissue. Pulp protection is fundamental to crown provision. Non-vital or pulpally involved teeth that are not already filled also usually make for a relatively straightforward planning decision, as the infection clearly needs to be managed. There are very few, if any, circumstances where a crown should be placed over a tooth with an infected pulp where no attempt at endodontic treatment has been made.

The greatest clinical quandary arises with teeth that have already been root treated, but without a long-term resolution of the pathology, or where the technical quality of the root filling is dubious. Data from the UK suggest that most root treated teeth would actually fall into the latter category.[2,8,9] Endodontics can be difficult enough at first attempt, but a technically satisfactory result is even more difficult where an unsatisfactory attempt has already been made. Re-treatment decisions have to be made on a

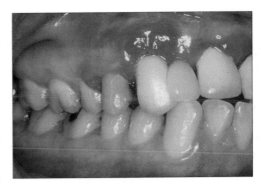

Fig. 19 'gingival inflammation related to anterior crown margins'

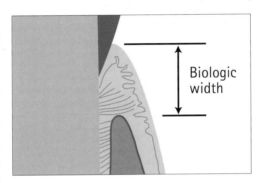

Fig. 20 'biologic width'

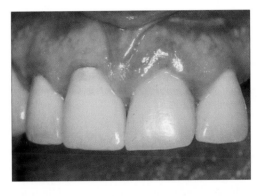

Fig. 21 'biologic width encroachment'

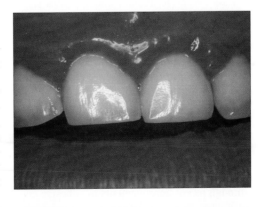

Fig. 22 'subgingival margins and gingival inflammation'

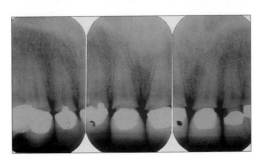

Fig. 23 'poorly fitting anterior crowns resulting from inaccurate impressions'

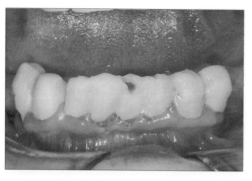

Fig. 24 'poor temporisation'

tooth-by-tooth basis and will be influenced by your own skill as an endodontist, or the access to a specialist in this demanding discipline. These are the foundations though, and you would think twice before replacing a roof where there is dry rot in the rafters.

Part 4 of the series covers these issues in some detail, including ways of restoring the core of the tooth using the root canal for retention.

Is the tooth itself strong enough to receive and retain a crown?

A number of basic factors should be considered before preparing any tooth for a crown. The extent of an existing restoration will influence the strength of the remaining tooth tissue and adequate retention of an extensive restoration is important to prevent complete coronal breakdown, even with a crown in place. The patient who enters the surgery with a crown containing an inadequate core or fractured tooth (usually neatly wrapped in tissue paper) is unfortunately a common scenario.

A properly constructed core with appropriate retentive features on a sound, disease free tooth can usually prevent this situation. Previous endodontic treatment will also affect the strength of the remaining tooth tissue, particularly where access cavities and coronal destruction are extensive. Parts 4 and 7 in this series cover the issues of core build up in detail, but decisions about the need for a core are an integral part of the planning process.

Will the preparation be retentive enough?

Adequate clinical crown height is a critical factor for the retention of full coronal restorations. Unless you plan to increase the occlusal vertical dimension, teeth with short clinical crowns will be even shorter and potentially very unretentive following crown preparation. This is particularly relevant for the restoration of worn teeth and although recent improvements in adhesive dentistry have increased the options for enhancing retention, mechanical retention by appropriate tooth preparation remains essential for predictable success and longevity of coronal restorations. Specific design features to optimise retention as well as crown lengthening will be covered in Part 8 in this series.

Is there enough space for my restoration?

Tooth wear not only results in problems of retention but also in providing adequate occlusal space for your restoration. As we have just discussed increasing the occlusal vertical dimension can obviate the need for occlusal reduction on the preparation and can provide additional length that will improve retention, and often allows for improved aesthetics as well. Clearly, such an approach will involve extensive restorations and could involve the whole of one or both arches. However other strategies are available to make space.

The easiest way to provide sufficient clearance is to reduce the height of the opposing tooth, but whilst simple, this is often not advisable. Another approach, which is conservative of tooth tissue, is to make a local temporary increase in vertical dimension to promote axial orthodontic tooth movements (eg a Dahl appliance, or an occlusal composite build-up). The patient needs to be informed that the required tooth movements can take several months and you have to be careful to ensure that the built-up teeth are being loaded axially. This approach is being used increasingly on supra-occluding restorations by at least one centre.[10]

Occasionally space can be created anteriorly by adjusting the posterior teeth to eliminate deflective contacts, which repositions the mandible distally.

None of the above options should be undertaken lightly, but a detailed consideration falls outside the remit of this series. All of these techniques are well described in a recent article by Dyer et al. (2001), which provides a useful introduction to contemporary methods of managing space and problems of reduced crown height.[11]

What next? The staged treatment plan

Although a clear vision of the finished treatment is indispensable at the outset we sometimes find that the initial plan is inappropriate and changes have to be made. This is because one or other of the questions listed above are answered in a different way from the way you expected. Perhaps hygiene continues to be a problem, or perhaps it improves unexpectedly, maybe the core breaks down or you find a root crack during endodontics. It pays to keep flexible, and to review the plan at key stages as you progress. Failure to do this can leave you committed to a course of action which may become increasingly difficult to sustain and which may fail much sooner than anticipated.

It is always worth discussing the alternative treatment options with your patient before starting work. In this way a change of plan can be made at an early stage rather than carrying on regardless and subsequently having to explain an expensive failure later. Anticipating problems is one of the key skills of the experienced restorative dentist and contingency planning is an essential element of any complex treatment plan.

Conclusion

In the course of this article we have posed seven key questions to ask yourself before you finally plan treatment and pick up a handpiece. Success with crowns and other extra-coronal restorations depends on many interacting factors; technical issues related to tooth preparation, the relationship with the pulp and periodontal tissues and occlusion have been introduced and will be covered in greater detail later in this series. However, the emphasis has been on planning for the future rather than providing a short-term fix for single teeth in isolation. The needs and expectations of the patient are key elements in the treatment planning process as is the importance of minimising further damage to the dentition and reducing the risk of disease in the future. These essential factors could perhaps be summarised in one overriding question before embarking on a course of treatment : 'will this patient's oral health be better off when I have finished?'. If there are any doubts about the answer to this question, the plan should be modified and an alternative approach considered.

1. Kelly M, Steele J, Nuttall N, Bradnock G, Morris J, Nunn J, Pine C, Pitts N, Treasure E, White D. *Adult Dental Health Survey: Oral Health in the United Kingdom in 1998.* (2000) London: TSO.

2. Saunders W P, Saunders E M. Prevalence of periapical pathoses associated with crowned teeth in a Scottish sub-population. *Br Dent J* 1998; **185:** 137-140.

3. Valderhaug A, Jokstad, Ambjornsen E, Norheim P W. Assessment of the periapical and clinical status of crowned teeth over 25 years. *J Dent* 1997; **25:** 97-105.

4. Bergenholtz G. Iatrogenic injury to the pulp in dental procedures: Aspects of pathogenesis, management and preventive measures. *Int Dent J* 1991; **41:** 99-110.

5. Steele J G, Sheiham A, Marcenes W, Fay N, Walls A W G. Clinical behavioural risk indicators for root caries in older people. *Gerodontol* 2001; **18:** 95-101.

6. Steele J G, Walls A W G, Murray J J. Partial dentures as an independent indicator of root caries risk in a group of older adults. *Gerodontol* 1998; **14:** 67-74.

7. Locker D. Incidence of root caries in an older Canadian Population. *Comm Dent Oral Epidemiol* 1996; **24:** 403-407.

8. Dummer P M H. *The quality of root canal treatment provided by General dental Services working within the general dental services of England and Wales.* Part 1. *Dent Profile* 1997; **17:** 1-5.

9. Dummer P M H. The quality of root canal treatment provided by General dental Services working within the general dental services of England and Wales. Part 2. *Dent Profile* 1998; **19:** 8-10.

10. Gough M B, Setchell D J. A retrospective study of 50 treatments using an appliance to produce localised occlusal space by relative axial tooth movement. *Br Dent J* 1999; **187:** 134-139.

11. Dyer K, Ibbetson R, Grey N. A question of space: Options for the restorative management of worn teeth. *Dent Update* 2001; **28:** 118-123.

IN BRIEF

- A consideration of the impact of crowning on the dental pulp, and the special issues involved in crowning root-treated teeth.
- The damaging effects of crown preparation.
- Assessment and preparation of root-treated and non root-treated teeth to minimize endodontic complications.
- Special considerations in the temporisation and restoration of root-treated teeth.

Crowns and other extra-coronal restorations: Endodontic considerations: the pulp, the root-treated tooth and the crown

J. M. Whitworth[1] A. W. G. Walls[2] and R. W. Wassell[3]

Endodontic considerations is the fourth in the series on crowns and other extra-coronal restorations. This article focuses strongly on contemporary biological principles, and is not intended to provide a comprehensive review of commercially available materials and techniques. Principles are illustrated in a variety of clinical case scenarios.

[1]Senior Lecturer,
[2]Professor,
[3]Senior Lecturer in Restorative Dentistry,
Department of Restorative Dentistry,
The Dental School, Framlington Place,
Newcastle upon Tyne NE2 4BW
*Correspondence to: Dr J. M. Whitworth
E-mail: j.m.whitworth@ncl.ac.uk

Crowns should not be made without consideration of the teeth which lay the foundations for them. In this article, important principles are outlined for the assessment of root-treated and non root-treated teeth before crowning, avoiding endodontic complications during crown fabrication, and special considerations in the temporisation and restoration of root-treated teeth.

Pulp morbidity in crowned teeth

Dental pulp is the highly vascular, richly innervated soft tissue structure whose principal role is tooth formation. But even after teeth are erupted into the mouth and fully formed, the dental pulp is not a redundant organ. Pulp tissue retains the important function of supporting its secretory odontoblasts which lay down reparative dentine in defensive response to dental injuries throughout life. There is also some evidence that the pulp may be involved in a pressure-receptive function, limiting the possibility of damaging functional overload on teeth.[1]

If this were not sufficient justification to preserve healthy pulps, then the desire to do patients no harm and to avoid the pain, swelling and suffering which often accompanies the injury and demise of a pulp surely must be.

An insulating coverage of dentine and an impervious layer of enamel protect the pulps of healthy, intact teeth from injury. Crown preparation places the pulp at risk in a number of ways. High speed stripping of hard tissue poses the threat of pulpal overheating, with disturbance of microcirculation, vascular stasis, thrombosis, reduced blood flow and internal bleeding.[2] It also

opens a multitude of dentinal tubules that communicate directly with the pulp. The deeper the dentine is cut, the more permeable it is,[3] and the more vulnerable the pulp becomes to chemical, physical and microbial irritants. The microbial threat presented by the oral flora is by far the most serious, and is capable of heralding intense inflammatory changes, with micro-abscess formation and progressive pulpal necrosis.[4,5]

Although the pulp shows considerable resilience and is often capable of recovering from irritation, the injuries induced can become significant in the long term.[5] Scarring as a result of inflammation and repair interferes with the nervous and vascular supply to the tissue[6] and jeopardises its resistance to further insult. It is important in this respect to recognise that crowns are rarely made for pristine, intact teeth. Rather, they are made to protect and restore teeth which have been damaged by wear, trauma, or cycles of caries and repair. After a lifetime of cumulative insult, crown preparation can be the final straw, bringing pulpal breakdown (Fig. 1a), and the need for root canal treatment.[7]

It is uncertain how many teeth lose vitality as a direct consequence of crown preparation. Bergenholtz and Nyman's[8] much quoted study showed that 9% of crowned teeth, compared with only 2% of uncrowned controls lost vitality during long-term review. None of this was attributable to caries or other obvious causes, but the crowned teeth in this study did have advanced periodontal destruction, and were involved in extensive, cross-arch bridgework.

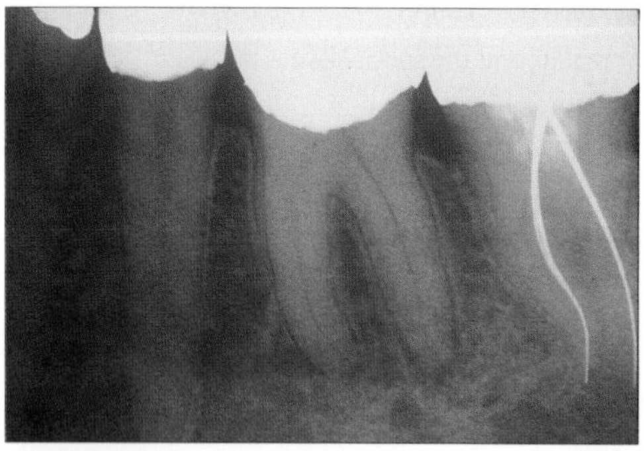

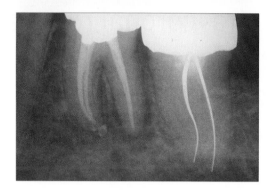

Fig. 1a Pulpal breakdown and acute apical periodontitis affecting a recently crowned mandibular first molar

Fig. 1b Root-treatment completed through the crown without serious damage

A more realistic estimation may be in the order of 4–8% in the 10 years following active treatment.[10-13] This estimation does, however, assume that efforts were made to identify and manage all obvious pulpal pathosis before crowns were made; an assumption that cannot always be taken for granted in practice and which increases the likely incidence of unexpected endodontic problems that need attention at a later date.

The dangers of root-treating crowned teeth

Extra-coronal restorations do not rule out root-treatment or retreatment (Fig. 1b), but it should be noted that working through a crown is always more difficult, and that damage can be done.

Just piercing the glaze of a porcelain crown dramatically reduces its strength,[14] whilst cutting through a metal ceramic crown can weaken the porcelain bond and predispose to fracture. Vibration can disturb the cement lute of a casting and predispose leakage or loss, whilst rubber-dam clamps may crack and pit cervical porcelain[15] and occasionally cause a crown to debond.

Once through the crown, the search for the pulp can be hazardous. Metal copings and cores obscure the pulp and prevent its location and assessment from preoperative radiographs. The alignment and rotation of the crown may also not correspond to the underlying tooth, causing loss of orientation and misdirected cutting. Added to this, problems are compounded by limited entry of light and poor visibility.

All of this can leave the operator severely weakening the core and vertical walls of the tooth in search for the pulp chamber and canal

Extrapolation to the case of uncomplicated, single crowns is therefore difficult.

Even higher levels of pulp death were recorded by Felton et al.,[9] where 13.3% of teeth restored with full coverage crowns, compared with 0.5% of unrestored controls lost vitality during the 3–30 year review period. But it was not possible to derive from this report how many teeth had suffered further pulpal insult, such as recurrent caries, which may have artificially inflated the adverse effects reported.

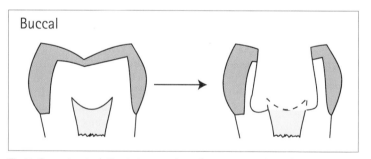

Buccal

Fig. 2a Overcut and misdirected access through a crown grossly weakens the vertical walls of the preparation

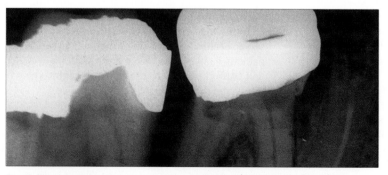

Fig. 2b Disorientated by the presence of a crown which had modestly realigned the tooth, the access cavity into this lower molar completely bypassed the pulp chamber to the mesial and lingual. There were no less than five separate perforations

openings (Fig. 2a). Catastrophic errors such as perforation are also possible (Fig. 2b).

Of equal importance is the damage that can be done to patient confidence and trust if a recently crowned tooth becomes troublesome and has to be accessed or the restoration removed for endodontic treatment.[16] As the complexity of the crown and bridgework increases, so the consequences become more serious. Replacing a single crown damaged during access is one matter; replacing a large bridge which has suffered irreparable damage to one of its abutments is quite another.

It is certain that a small number of teeth will always develop unexpected endodontic problems after crowning,[11] but it is also certain that many such instances can be avoided by careful preoperative workup.

PREVENTATIVE ENDONDONTICS — AVOIDING THE AVOIDABLE

All teeth scheduled to be crowned, whether they are presumed to have healthy pulps or previously root-treated should be thoroughly assessed at the planning stage. In this way, potential endodontic problems can be identified and addressed and future embarrassment and trauma kept to a minimum.

Teeth presumed to have healthy pulps

Pulps cannot be visualised directly to assess their health. Neither is there a single test which will reliably deliver this information in all circumstances. We rely therefore on a combination of fairly crude methods, including pain history, clinical examination, special tests and radiographs to build a picture of pulp status. All teeth due to be crowned should be tested systematically to give as clear a picture as possible.

Pain history

A brief pain history reveals areas of the mouth sensitive to hot, cold or sweet, and teeth sensitive to chewing pressure, which require further examination. Review of the case notes may identify teeth with a history of trauma, pulpal exposure or pulpitic symptoms. But this is not enough. Despite textbook accounts of classical toothaches, most injured pulps die quietly, and it is also known that pulpal pain is poorly localised. The absence of reported symptoms is therefore not proof of health, and further examination is needed to identify inflamed and necrotic pulps in need of treatment.

Clinical examination

Indications of pulp condition may come from the identification of caries, large or leaking restorations, non-carious tooth tissue loss and traumatic injury. Inspection and palpation of soft tissues overlying the apices of teeth to be crowned may reveal signs of endodontic pathosis, including swelling, redness and discharging fistulae. Non-vital teeth may appear slightly darker than their neighbours, and periapically

involved teeth may be tender to biting pressure or gentle percussion.

Special tests

Characteristically, pulpal symptoms are difficult for patients to localise, and require systematic provocation and reproduction to identify the offending tooth with certainty. If sensitivity is reported to hot or cold, the teeth should be challenged with that stimulus. Cold can be applied with an ethyl chloride soaked cotton pledget, though ice sticks or proprietary refrigerants such as Endo-Frost (Reoko) can give a more profound cold challenge to stimulate the pulps of old or heavily restored teeth. Heat can be applied with a stick of warm gutta percha 'temporary stopping', taking care to coat the tooth first with petroleum jelly to prevent the hot material from adhering. Electronic touch and heat instruments used in thermoplastic gutta percha filling techniques can also be used to deliver a known and reproducible thermal challenge.

As a general rule, thermal tests are more discriminating of pulp condition than electrical.[17] They should be repeated, and contralateral and adjacent teeth tested for reference. An exaggerated and lingering response may indicate irreversible pulpal inflammation, whilst a consistent absence of response may suggest pulp necrosis.

Pulp sensitivity tests are essential in pre-operative assessment, but their results should not be taken in isolation, and should always be interpreted with caution.

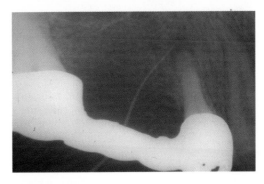

Fig. 3 A gutta percha point inserted into a discharging fistula locates its source at the apex of the premolar bridge abutment

Radiographs

Periapical radiographs should be of diagnostic quality and taken by a paralleling technique. If there is a discharging fistula, a gutta percha cone size 25 or 30 should be inserted to source the infectious focus (Fig. 3). More than one film, taken at different angles, may be needed to visualise all roots and all root canals, and should be examined for apical and lateral lesions of endodontic origin. If root-treatment is indicated, an assessment should be made of the degree of difficulty this presents, and whether a predictable, quality result is likely.

The size of a healthy, vital pulp should also be noted, especially if the reason for the crown is to realign the tooth. Heavy tooth reduction in such cases may result in embarrassing unexpected pulpal exposure.

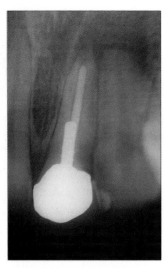

Fig. 4 Pain and swelling associated with a tooth which was recently crowned without revising the unsatisfactory endodontic foundation

Fig. 5 A technically satisfactory root-filling exposed to the mouth through defective restoration margins. Oral microbes will rapidly invade the canal system and compromise the root-treatment. Endodontic retreatment should be considered before a new crown is made

Previously root-treated teeth

Previously root-treated teeth also need critical appraisal before crowning.

Clinical signs and symptoms of endodontic failure obviously demand endodontic retreatment or surgical revision before a crown is made, but even in the absence of symptoms, technically inadequate, short or poorly condensed root fillings (Fig. 4) do not represent predictable foundations and should be revised. Even if the resultant root filling is not better extended, recleaning the canal system can only improve the internal environment of the tooth, and make a better foundation for restoration.

A further group of unreliable teeth is those where the root filling has been open to the mouth through defective restoration margins or restoration loss (Fig. 5). Saliva and micro-organisms migrate quickly alongside exposed root fillings,[18] and whilst firm rules are difficult to make, it is probably wise to revise all root fillings that have been exposed to the mouth for more than a month, even if they appear technically satisfactory on radiographs. The appearance of the film in such cases denies the biological status of the canal system.

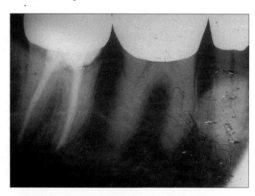

Treatment planning and guidelines

Teeth identified as having necrotic pulps, or showing signs of irreversible pulpal inflammation should be root-treated before crowns are prepared. Elective root-canal treatment should also be planned for teeth whose pulps are at serious risk of exposure during crown preparation, and for teeth that cannot be restored without using the pulp chamber and root canals for retention and support. Pulps accidentally exposed during crown preparation should not be capped; root canal therapy should proceed.

Technically inadequate root fillings, and root fillings which have been exposed to the mouth, should be replaced before crowning. This option is always preferable to retreatment or corrective surgery after the event. Decisiveness is also called for in the case of teeth which are unrestorable, or which are of very poor prognosis. Procrastination rarely rewards the practitioner and such teeth should be planned for extraction.

If there is doubt in a complex case over diagnosis, or the ability of the practitioner to lay a reliable endodontic foundation, referral for a specialist opinion should be considered.

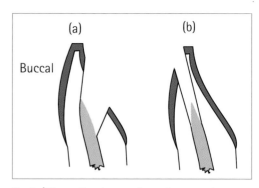

Fig. 6 a) Conventional access does not compromise aesthetics, but sacrifices much lingual tissue.
b) Labial/incisal access preserves tissue in teeth scheduled to be crowned. The access can be aesthetically temporised with composite resin

Detailed accounts of contemporary root-treatment and retreatment techniques are beyond the scope of this article, and readers are referred to standard texts.[19,20] However, important guiding principles should be stated. Root-treatment or retreatment should sacrifice a minimum of structurally important tooth tissue, which is compatible with quality care. Access cavities should not be over-cut and root canals should not be over-flared; to do so simply risks weakening the tooth further. Anterior teeth may in fact be best accessed though the incisal and labial surfaces to preserve tissue[21] (Fig. 6).

Posterior teeth may be reduced out of occlusion at the start of treatment to minimise the risk from damaging wedging forces splitting the accessed tooth, and the additional support of a well-fitting orthodontic band cemented with glass-ionomer cement may be considered for badly broken-down and vulnerable teeth (Fig. 7).

After root-treatment is complete, provisional restorations should be in place for the minimum time possible and should seal against the ingress of saliva and micro-organisms to the canal system, which will predispose failure. Temporary restorations in place for any time should also provide the necessary protection and support to prevent tooth fracture. Further consideration will be given later to the temporisation and restoration of root-treated teeth.

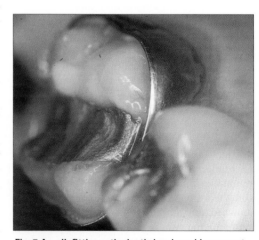

Fig. 7 A well-fitting orthodontic band provides support and protection for a vulnerable posterior tooth

MINIMISING DAMAGE TO TEETH WITH HEALTHY PULPS

Having now identified and treated those teeth with inflamed, necrotic or at risk pulps, the remaining teeth should be treated with all respect to preserve their pulps in health. Frictional heat generated during crown preparation should be strictly controlled. Although dentine is a good thermal insulator, damaging rises in temperature can occur, especially in preparations involving substantial tissue removal. High volume, well focused water-cooling should be used at all times,[22,23] and cutting strokes should be intermittent and light.

Open dentinal tubules should also be managed with care and respect. Cut dentine should not be over-dried with the 3 in 1 syringe, and smear plugs should not be removed by the careless application of acidic astringents used in gingival haemorrhage control.

Bacteria and their metabolic by-products are the greatest danger to pulp health,[24,25] and it behoves the practitioner to ensure that temporary and permanent crowns fit accurately and provide the best possible marginal seal. The pre-sealing of dentine with a resin-bonding agent may be a means of reducing dentine permeability and enhancing pulp protection,[26] though there are few published data to date which specifically demonstrate the effectiveness of this action in preserving the pulps of crown-prepared teeth.

RESTORATION OF THE ROOT-TREATED TOOTH

General considerations

Root-treated teeth are in a vulnerable state until they are permanently restored.

The risks they face fall into two major categories:

1. Fracture of remaining tooth tissue
2. Reinfection of the root canal from the mouth

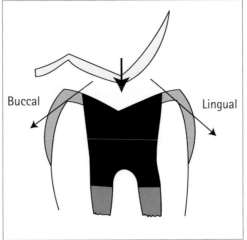
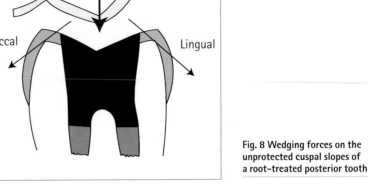

Fig. 8 Wedging forces on the unprotected cuspal slopes of a root-treated posterior tooth

These two considerations underpin the approach to temporising and restoring all root-treated teeth.

Protecting root-treated teeth from fracture

It is widely held that root-treated teeth are brittle. Historically, this has been attributed to desiccation, or other physical changes in the dentine of pulpless teeth, which reduce its toughness.

More recently, it has been recognised that the key change is the loss of structural tissue which is capable of holding the tooth together under functional load. This is especially so for posterior teeth, where wedging forces come to bear (Fig. 8). Conservative access preparation in an otherwise sound tooth may not be especially damaging, but endodontic access in combination with the earlier loss of one or both marginal ridges leaves the tooth at serious risk, even if it was reduced from direct occlusal contact before endodontic treatment began.

For this reason, some form of cuspal coverage should always be provided for root-treated posterior teeth,[27] unless the endodontic access is the

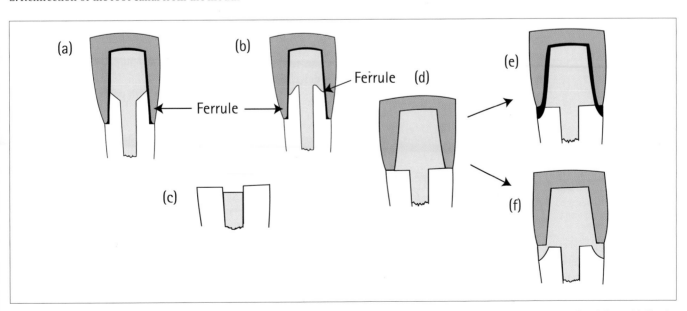

Fig. 9 The development of protective ferrules for anterior teeth: a) Moderate loss of tooth tissue — the post and core provide no protection, a ferrule is provided by the crown; b) Moderate loss of tooth tissue — bevelling of the residual tooth tissue allows the core as well as the crown to provide protective ferrules; c) Decoronated, root-treated anterior tooth which is vulnerable to fracture and requires protection; d) No protective ferrule provided by the core, or by the crown; e) No protection provided by the core, but the crown extends onto tooth and provides a protective ferrule; and f) Protective ferrule provided by a cast post and diaphragm

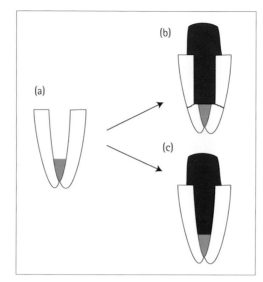

Figure 10 a) Wide and tapered root canal. b) Preparation for a parallel post removes more tissue and weakens the root further. Stresses are also concentrated at the sharp angles of the post terminus. c) Custom cast metal post requires little or no further loss of tissue

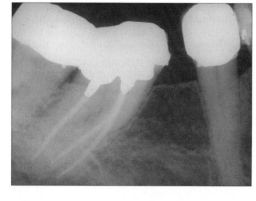

Fig. 11 Canal entrances and pulp chamber anatomy used to retain an all amalgam core in a molar. Composite resin may be used in a similar way for anterior teeth

rior teeth. For such teeth ferrules should be incorporated as routine.

Posts: a means of protecting teeth from fracture?

Another popular misconception is that the cementation of a metallic post in a root-treated tooth provides reinforcement. In reality, the post offers no reinforcement, and dentine removal to accommodate it may in fact weaken the tooth further and create an area of stress concentration at the terminus of the post channel (Fig. 10).

The chief function of a post is to retain the core. If adequate retention for the core can be derived from the use of natural undercuts in the pulp chamber and canal entrances (Fig. 11), then a post should not be used.

If a post really is required, then consideration should be given to how it can provide retention for the core without weakening or stressing the tooth, or compromising the effectiveness of the root filling.

Practitioners are not short of choice in post selection, and it is certainly beyond the scope of this article to consider the many systems available in any detail. A review of commercially available systems by Edmunds and Dummer[29–32] ran to no less than four articles, and new systems continue to appear.

The literature contains many *in vitro* reports of post performance and failure characteristics, but as in many other areas of dentistry, well-controlled clinical studies are few and far between. Objective judgements cannot therefore be made on the performance of many of the available post systems, though certain principal considerations can be derived.

It is likely that many post systems will provide satisfactory retention for the coronal restoration, but the potential cost of enhancing retention should be considered. Dentists should perhaps focus less on factors which maximise retention and more on factors that affect resistance to root fracture,[27] ie the preservation and protection of tooth tissue, and the avoidance of stressing restoration components.

Avoiding problems with posts

Post length

There is little doubt that long posts are more retentive than short posts. Endodontic posts should therefore be as long as possible, and it is important to note that this is achieved not only by extending the post apically, but also by preserving tooth tissue coronally (Fig. 12). There is no place for the decoronating 'rooftop' preparation in the restoration of root-filled teeth. This is particularly so when evidence suggests that at least 4–5 mm of gutta percha should remain apically to ensure that the seal of the root filling is not compromised.[11,33]

Retaining coronal dentine also allows for wrap-around coverage by the subsequent crown, which provides the essential 'ferrule effect' discussed earlier (Fig. 12c).

only coronal tissue loss, and there are no damaging functional or parafunctional loads on the tooth.

Incisors and canines are spared the wedging cuspal deflections of posterior teeth, but they too can suffer longitudinal fracture if significant tooth tissue has been lost, and a protective ferrule is not incorporated into the coronal restoration. A ferrule is a band of metal which totally encircles the tooth, extending 1–2 mm onto sound tooth tissue to guard against longitudinal fracture.[28] Figure 9 shows examples of ferrules for moderately and severely broken down ante-

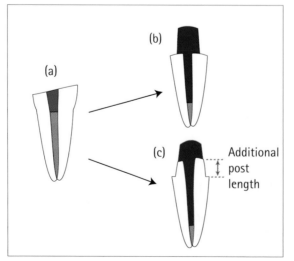

Fig. 12 a) Fractured and root-treated incisor to be restored with a post retained crown. b) Rooftop preparation damagingly removes all remaining coronal tooth tissue, and may compromise the ability to create a protective ferrule. c) Conservative preparation preserves tooth tissue, lengthens the post, and allows the development of protective ferrules

Additional post length

Post shape

All other factors being equal, parallel-sided posts, such as the Parapost (Fig. 13) are more retentive than tapered posts.[34] However, the preparation of a parallel-sided post channel, and subsequent cementation of a square-ended parallel post may produce increased stress in the narrow and tapering root-end[35] (Fig. 14a) and predispose to root fracture. Systems, which are bevelled apically may therefore be preferred (Fig. 14b). But once again, the preservation of tooth tissue is important to the long-term integrity of the tooth, and tissue should not be sacrificed in order to create a parallel-sided post channel if a well-adapted tapered post can be placed with less sacrifice of dentine.

Tapered posts such as the PD system have a good record of clinical success.[36] Concerns have often been raised over the generation of wedging stresses by tapered (including customised cast) posts, and the tendency to promote root fracture. However, such forces are not active in the same way as those generated by self-tapping screw systems, and it may be that many cases of root fracture associated with tapered posts reflect the type of cases in which such posts are often used, ie the wide, thin-walled tapered canal. Again, the importance of providing a protective coronal ferrule cannot be over-emphasised.

In their study of parallel versus tapered post systems, Torbjornet *et al.*[34] noted that in fact the type of post may be of minimal importance to the risk of root fracture if the tooth is covered by a complete crown with a good ferrule effect at the crown margin area. Their comments were not, however, directed to posts involving active methods of retention.

Customised cast posts are especially versatile and can often be fabricated with the minimum of additional canal preparation. Such posts have a strong history of clinical success[28,37] especially once again when a coronal ferrule is provided.

In summary, parallel-sided posts are preferred to tapered posts, but each case should be carefully considered on its merits, and dentine should not be unnecessarily sacrificed to dogmatically satisfy the desire to place a moderately more retentive parallel post.

Surface characteristics: threaded versus non-threaded posts

There is little doubt from the literature that threaded post systems offer the maximum mechanical retention. But the retention they provide is often by active engagement of elastic dentine, producing stress concentration around the threads, and increasing the risk of root fracture.[38] This is especially so if posts are self-tapping, and is amplified if the post also has a wedge-like, tapered design.

Popular commercial threaded posts include:

- Radix Anker (Fig. 15)
- Dentatus (Fig. 16)
- Kurer Anchor (Fig. 17)

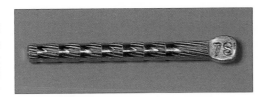

Fig. 13 Parapost — parallel, serrated post

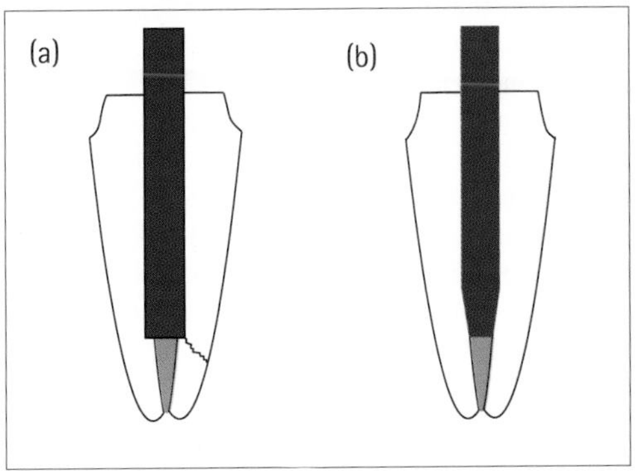

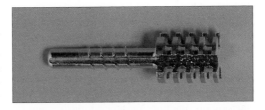

Fig. 14 a) Stress concentration at the base of a parallel post preparation. b) Reduced stress concentration with a chamfered tip

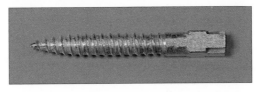

Fig. 15: Radix Anker — parallel, self-tapping or pre-tapped post

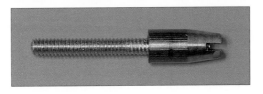

Fig. 16 Dentatus screw — tapered, self-tapping post

Fig. 17 Kurer Anchor — parallel, threaded post for which the root canal is pre-tapped

Concerns have been expressed about all threaded post systems, and it is notable that most manufacturers now recommend that the post is used first to cut a thread, and is then removed and reinserted with cement, or is simply derotated a quarter turn to reduce stresses which are generated during initial insertion. The Kurer post system, in which the canal is first tapped before post insertion, is probably the least stressing of threaded post systems. Another method of limiting stress is seen in the Flexipost, which incorporates a split-pin mechanism, the split pin collapsing upon itself as the post is inserted to reduce pressure on the canal walls.[39]

Generally speaking, threaded posts are not preferred and Meta analysis of the limited clinical evidence available suggests that their performance is inferior to that of customised cast posts.[37] If enhanced retention is required in a special situation, then threaded posts are no longer the only option. Increasingly, resin-bonding agents may be employed with serrated, and preferably sandblasted metal or fibre posts, reducing the potential for stress, and enhancing the possibility of developing an hermetic coronal seal.[28]

Minimising danger during post space preparation

Ideally, post space preparation is completed at the appointment when the root canal is filled. At this time, the practitioner is most familiar with the canal system and reference points. He is also able to make post space with the rubber dam in place to minimise microbial entry, and can further condense the apical segment of the root filling after the coronal gutta percha has been removed. Gutta percha removal and post channel preparation should not be undertaken in a single act with the aggressive end-cutting twist drills provided with proprietary post systems. To do so is to risk losing alignment and perforating the root for the sake of a few seconds of time. Gutta percha should first be removed to the predetermined length using burs with non-cutting tips (eg Gates Glidden) or with hot instruments before the channel is shaped and enlarged progressively with measured twist drills.

Guarding against coronal microleakage

Coronal microleakage is a major cause of endodontic failure.[40] Saliva and organisms from the mouth migrate rapidly alongside poorly adapted restorations and even root fillings which appear well condensed.[18] The periradicular tissues will be inflamed by such reinfection and the reactivation of micro-organisms lying dormant after initial treatment. A well sealing coronal restoration is critical therefore to endodontic success, and it is again stressed that this applies as strongly to temporary restorations as it does to permanent ones. Posterior teeth can be temporised with cuspal-coverage amalgam restorations, which will prove durable and well sealing for many months or years. But the same cannot be said for anterior temporary post crowns, which should be in place for the minimum time possible.

Restorations should be well adapted, and every use should be made of modern adhesive systems in an effort to control salivary entry.

TREATMENT GUIDELINES

In summary, the guiding principles in restoring root-treated teeth are:

1. Preserve as much tooth tissue as possible
2. If a post is needed make sure it is long enough to be retentive and sufficiently strong to resist distortion
3. Avoid twist drills for the removal of gutta percha
4. Avoid active restorations or restoration components which induce internal stresses
5. Provide the necessary coronal coverage for protection
6. Strive for the best possible fluid and bacteria-tight seal

These principles will now be illustrated for a variety of restorative scenarios.

Minimal loss of coronal tissue

Incisors and canines which have lost tissue during access preparation, in addition to tissue loss caused by caries in one or both proximal surfaces can often be restored to satisfactory long-term function and aesthetics with dentine and enamel-bonded composite resin. Gutta percha should be cleared from the interior of the crown with hot instruments or Gates Glidden drills. Powerful organic solvents such as chloroform or halothane are not recommended in post channel preparation, as it is impossible to control their advance into the root canal where they can rapidly dissolve gutta percha and sealer at a deeper level than anticipated. All traces of sealer should be removed from the coronal tissues to prevent later discolouration. Concerns have been expressed about zinc oxide-eugenol sealers in particular, traces of which may interfere with the polymerisation of restorative resins. Alcohol rapidly sequesters excess eugenol and is not known to threaten the integrity of gutta percha root fillings. It may be wise to rinse the pulp chamber with alcohol to remove traces of eugenol before attempting to bond.[41]

Premolars and molars with only minimal access cavities and no other coronal tissue loss can be restored with amalgam or composite resin in combination with a resin bonding system to enhance the marginal seal. The restorative material should be extended 2–3 mm into canal entrances by carefully removing root filling material with hot instruments or Gates Glidden drills. However, large Gates should not be extended deeply into canals with the risk of unnecessary dentine removal, and even strip perforation. The first increments of core material should be packed with a long, narrow plugger (eg Mortensen Condenser) to ensure good adaptation into these retentive features.

Moderate loss of tooth tissue

Advances in bonding technology and improvements in the physical and aesthetic properties of composite resins continue to increase the potential for simple, plastic restoration of anterior teeth. Depending upon aesthetic and functional demands, root-treated teeth with proximal and incisal tissue loss, in addition to the access cavity may often be restored without the need for a crown. Bonding composite resin soon after completion of the root filling has the added advantage of securing an early, hermetic seal against coronal microleakage.

It is impossible in this context to lay down firm rules on the precise degree of tissue loss that can be successfully restored in this non-destructive way. But it should also be noted that teeth restored with simple plastic restorations can always be revisited at a later stage for a more advanced and destructive restoration if the need arises.

Anterior teeth, which have some coronal tissue remaining, but where this is considered insufficient for long-term restoration with composite resin, either on functional or aesthetic grounds, require core build-up and a crown. The core may not always need a post for retention.

Gutta percha and sealer are first cleared from the crown and coronal 2–3 mm of the root canal. The remaining coronal tooth tissue is then prepared to receive a crown. Under no circumstances should the tooth be decoronated to create a 'rooftop' preparation (Fig.12a, b). Weak, undermined coronal tissue and spurs of tissue, which are taller than they are wide, should be reduced and the remaining, well-supported tissue bevelled. Every effort should be made to preserve as much coronal tissue as possible. If there is adequate retention and support available for the core material, then dentine-bonded composite is cured into the chamber and extended to complete the preparation coronally.

If tissue loss is more severe, then a post is required (Fig. 12c). This may either be cast, or prefabricated. Gutta percha is removed from the canal, leaving 4–5 mm of filling material apically. An initial path is made with hot instruments, or with Gates Glidden drills, numbers 2 and 3, which should be running at the maximum speed achievable with the slow speed handpiece to generate frictional heat which will soften the gutta percha and ease its removal without disturbing the apical root filling.[42] Having created a path, twist drills appropriate to the post system selected are used to enlarge and shape the channel. Excessive dentine should not be removed to accommodate snugly a preformed parallel post in a flared canal. In this situation, a tapered or customised cast post or a fibre post is often preferred.

Impressions may then be taken for the production of an indirectly constructed casting, or a direct pattern fabricated in the mouth. Metal castings have the advantage that features can be built in to provide a protective ferrule, and that they can be customised to minimise the need for dentine removal. The chief disadvantage of this approach is that the tooth will need temporisation with a temporary post crown, which is unlikely to provide an hermetic coronal seal during the time required to fabricate the post.[43]

For this reason, it may be preferable to restore the tooth immediately with a prefabricated post, and composite core.[43,44] An immediate, and permanent coronal seal is then secured. This benefit should be balanced in heavy loading situations with consideration of the strength of the core and the post-core interface. However the development of a ferrule by extending crown margins well onto sound tooth tissue should minimise the physical demands on the composite core. Such extension may be subgingival or involve a crown lengthening procedure or forced eruption to obtain supragingival margins.

Posterior teeth, which have lost one or both marginal ridges in addition to tooth loss for endodontic access, require cuspal coverage. Amalgam or composite cores can again often be retained without the need for posts. If a post is considered necessary, it should usually be placed in the straightest and most bulky root, commonly the distal in lower molars, and the palatal in upper molars. Premolar roots should be judged on their merits. Even if a post is placed, root-filling materials should always be removed from the entrances of other canals to provide supplementary retention for the core, and resistance to rotational torque.

A cuspal coverage restoration can then be prepared which fits the functional and aesthetic demands of the situation. This may be as conservative as a cast metal onlay, or three-quarter crown, or as extensive as a full-coverage metal or ceramo-metal crown (Fig. 18). Extracoronal restorations should be extended at least 1–2 mm onto sound tooth tissue to provide all-enveloping protection against fracture of the underlying tooth.

Adhesively retained plastic restorations cannot be relied upon as long-term internal splints. If there is no plan to crown a weakened posterior tooth, either because the root-treatment is on probation, or for financial reasons, then physical cuspal coverage and protection must be provided by the core material. Cusps adjacent to lost marginal ridges should be reduced in height by 3 mm and overlaid with dentine bonded amalgam or composite resin. Such restorations can provide cost-effective, durable service for many years.[45]

Extensive loss of tooth tissue

Teeth with little or no coronal tissue remaining require special measures to provide a protective ferrule. Again, surgical crown lengthening or forced eruption may be needed to allow the placement of restoration margins on sound tissue.

Anterior teeth may be prepared to receive a cast metal post and diaphragm (Fig. 19), with extension of the metal casting over the bevelled or chamfered margins of the root-face to provide

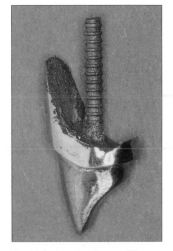

Fig. 19 Cast post and core with a diaphragm to cover and support a damaged incisor root

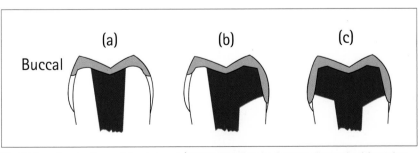

Fig. 18 Cuspal protection and development of protective ferrules for posterior teeth with varying amounts of tissue loss: a) Simple metal onlay, b) Three-quarter crown, c) Full coverage crown

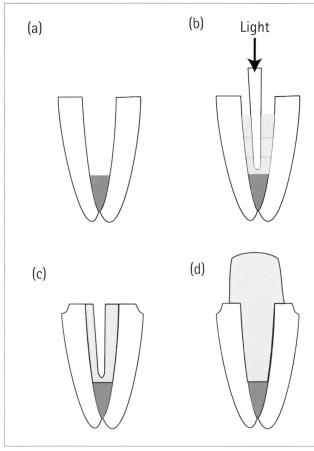

Fig. 20 Rehabilitation of a severely weakened tooth by relining with composite resin: a) Hollowed-out, fragile root; b) Incremental additions of composite cured with a light-transmitting post; c) Space for a conventional post within the composite resin 'reline'. Tooth margins prepared for the crown to provide a ferrule; and d) Continuous composite post and core takes advantage of the materials cohesive strength in thick section. Tooth margins prepared for the crown to provide a ferrule

Fig. 21 a) Metal post and core for a decoronated posterior tooth. The margins of the preparation are chamfered to provide a ferrule. The metal casting contains two short posts for the buccal roots. A separate wrought post will be inserted through it into the palatal root. b) The casting in place, with the wrought, parallel post cemented through it and into the palatal root

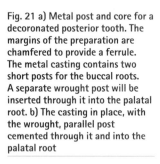
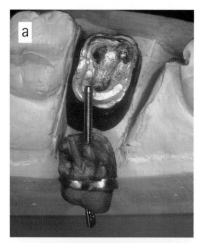
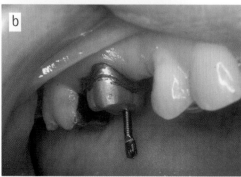

an effective ferrule. Alternatively, a conventional cast or prefabricated post and core may be placed, before constructing a crown with a metal collar extending 1–2 mm onto tooth tissue to afford the necessary protection.

Immature or hollowed-out roots can present special problems for rehabilitation. One method involves packing dentine bonded composite resin into the widened canal, and curing it in place with light-transmitting posts to effectively reline and internally splint the root (Fig. 20).[46] Alternatively, self-curing composite can be used. Conventional or fibre[44] posts may then be cemented into the 'relined' root before coronal core build-up, or advantage taken of the cohesive strength of composite in thick section to build a continuous mass of composite forming the post and core. The final crown should again incorporate a ferrule extending well onto sound tooth tissue for protection.

Posterior teeth which cannot be built up with post and adhesive-retained plastic materials may occasionally require the fabrication of a sectional casting. These restorations are difficult, exacting, and costly to manufacture and are testament to the engineering skills of practitioner and technician. Separate post and core elements with different paths of insertion that link on placement, or a single core unit with channels for multiple post placements at different angles may be manufactured (Fig. 21).

The extracoronal restoration should again be extended onto sound tooth tissue to provide a supporting ferrule for the underlying tooth.

In conclusion:

1. All teeth to be crowned should be carefully assessed as to their pulpal and endodontic status, and reliable foundations laid
2. Teeth with healthy pulps should be prepared and temporised with due care to preserve pulpal health
3. Root-treated teeth are at risk of fracture and of coronal microleakage. Control of these factors should underpin the design of all temporary and permanent restorations for such teeth.

1. Randlow K, Glanz P O. On cantilever loading of vital and non vital teeth: an experimental clinical study. *Acta Odontol Scand* 1986; **44:** 271-277.
2. Zach L. Pulp lability and repair: effect of restorative procedures. *Oral Surg* 1972; **33:** 111-121.
3. Pashley D H. Clinical considerations of microleakage. *J Endod* 1990; **16:** 70-77.
4. Cox C F, Subay R K, Suzuki S, Suzuki S H, Ostro E. Biocompatibility of various dental materials: pulp healing with a surface seal. *Int J Periodont Rest Dent* 1996; **16:** 241-251.
5. Bergenholtz G. Iatrogenic injury to the pulp in dental procedures: aspects of pathogenesis, management and preventive measures. *Int Dent J* 1991; **41:** 99-110.
6. Seltzer S, Bender I B. *The Dental Pulp.* 3rd Edition. pp324-348. Philadelphia: Lippincott, 1984.
7. Abou-Rass M. The stressed pulp condition: An endodontic-restorative diagnostic concept. *J Prosthet Dent* 1986; **48:** 264-267.
8. Bergenholtz G, Nyman S. Endodontic complications following periodontal and prosthetic treatment of patients with advanced periodontal disease. *J Periodontol* 1984; **55:** 63-68.
9. Felton D, Madison S, Kanoy E, Kantor M, Maryniuk G. Long

term effects of crown preparation on pulp vitality. *J Dent Res* 1989; **68** (special issue): 1009.

10. Landolt A, Lang N P. Erfolg und misserfolg bei extensionsbrucken. *Schweiz Monat Zahnmed* 1988; **98:** 239-44. [German with English abstract]

11. Reichen-Graden S, Lang N P. Periodontal and pulpal conditions of abutment teeth. *Schweiz Monat Zahnmed* 1989; **99:** 1381-1385.

12. Gonzalez G , Wier D J , Helm F , Marshall S J, Walker L, Stoffer W. *et al.* Incidence of endodontic treatment in teeth with full coverage restorations. *J Dent Res* 1991; **70** (special issue): 446.

13. Valderhaug J, Jokstad A, Ambjornsen E, Norheim P W. Assessment of the periapical and clinical status of crowned teeth over 25 years. *J Dent* 1997; **25:** 97-105.

14. McLean J W. *The Science and Art of Dental Materials.* Vol. 1. p 59. Chicago: Quintessence, 1979.

15. Madison S, Jordan R D, Krell K V. The effect of rubber dam retainers on porcelain fused-to-metal restorations. *J Endod* 1986; **12:** 183-186.

16. Dental Protection. Annual Report of the Board 1996; **8:** 22.

17. Cohen S. *In* Cohen S, Burns R C. (eds). *Pathways of the Pulp.* 6th edn. pp2-24. St Louis: Mosby, 1994.

18. Khayat A, Lee S J, Torabinejad M. Human saliva penetration of coronally unsealed obturated root canals. *J Endod* 1993; **19:** 458-461.

19. Walton R, Torabinejad M. *Principles and Practice of Endodontics.* 2nd edn. Baltimore: Saunders, 1996.

20. Pitt-Ford T R. *Harty's Endodontics in Clinical Practice.* 4th edn. Oxford: Wright, 1997.

21. Clements R E, Gilboe D B. Labial endodontic access opening for mandibular incisors: Endodontic and restorative considerations. *J Can Dent Assoc* 1991; **57:** 587-589.

22. Langeland K, Langeland L K. Pulp reactions to cavity and crown preparation. *Aust Dent J* 1970; **15:** 261-276.

23. Langeland K, Langeland L K. Cutting procedures with minimized trauma. *J Am Dent Assoc* 1968; **76:** 991-1005.

24. Bergenholtz G, Cox C, Loesche W J, Syed S A. Bacterial leakage around dental restorations: its effect on the dental pulp. *J Oral Pathol* 1982; **11:** 439-450.

25. Goldman M, Laosonthorn P, White R R. Microleakage: full crowns and the dental pulp. *J Endod* 1992; **18:** 473-475.

26. Cox C F, Suzuki S. Re-evaluating pulp protection: Calcium hydroxide liners vs. cohesive hybridization. *J Am Dent Assoc* 1994; **125:** 823-831.

27. Sorensen J A, Martinoff J T. Intracoronal reinforcement and coronal coverage: a study of endodontically treated teeth. *J Prosthet Dent* 1984; **51:** 781-784.

28. Morgano S M. Restoration of pulpless teeth: an application of traditional principles in present and future contexts. *J Prosth Dent* 1996; **75:** 375-380.

29. Edmunds D H, Dummer P M H. Root canal retained restorations: 1. General considerations and custom-made cast posts and cores. *Dent Update* 1990; June: 183-188.

30. Dummer P M H, Edmunds D H. Root canal retained restorations: 2. Prefabricated post and core systems — (i) Non-threaded posts. *Dent Update* 1990; July/August: 244-249.

31. Dummer P M H, Edmunds D H. Root canal retained restorations: 2. Prefabricated post and core systems — (ii) Threaded posts. *Dent Update* 1990; September: 286-289.

32. Edmunds D H, Dummer P M H. Root canal retained restorations revisited. *Dent Update* 1993; January/February: 14-19.

33. de Cleen M J H. The relationship between the root canal filling and post space preparation. *Int Endod J* 1993; **26:** 53-58.

34. Torbjorner A, Karlsson S, Odman P A. Survival rate and failure characteristics for two post designs. *J Prosthet Dent* 1995; **73:** 439-444.

35. Standlee J P, Caputo A A, Collard E W, Pollack M H. Analysis of stress distribution by endodontic posts. *Oral Surg* 1972; **33:** 952-960.

36. Weine F S, Wax A H, Wencus C S. Retrospective study of tapered smooth post systems in place for 10 years or more. *J Endodont* 1991; **17:** 293-297.

37. Creugers N H J, Mentink A G B, Kayser A F. An analysis of durability data on post and core restorations. *J Dent* 1993; **21:** 281-284.

38. Deutsch A S, Cavallari J, Musikant B L, *et al.* Root fracture and the design of prefabricated posts. *J Prosthet Dent* 1985; **53:** 637-640.

39. Cohen B I, Musikant B L, Deutsch A S. A 10-year literature review of a split-shanked threaded post. *Compend Cont Educ Dent* 1995: **16:** 630-631.

40. Saunders W P, Saunders E M. Coronal leakage as a cause of failure in root-canal therapy: a review. *Endod Dent Traumatol* 1994; **10:** 105-108.

41. Tjan A H L, Nemetz H. Effect of eugenol-containing endodontic sealer on retention of prefabricated posts luted with adhesive composite resin cement. *Quintessence Int* 1992; **23:** 839-844.

42. Haddix J E, Mattison G D, Shulmann C A *et al.* Post preparation techniques and their effect on the apical seal. *J Prosth Dent* 1990; **64:** 515-519.

43. Fox K, Gutteridge D L. An *in vitro* study of coronal microleakage in root-canal-treated teeth restored by the post and core technique. *Int Endod J* 1997; **30:** 361-368.

44. Ferrari M, Vichi A, Mannocci F, Mason PN. Retrospective study of the performance of fiber posts. *Amer J Dent* 2000; **13** (special issue): 9B-13B.

45. Nayyar A, Walton R E, Leonard L A. An amalgam coronal-radicular dowel and core technique for endodontically treated posterior teeth. *J Pros Dent* 1980; **43:** 511-515.

46. Saupe W A, Gluskin A H, Radke R A. A comparative study of fracture resistance between morphologic dowel and cores and a resin-reinforced dowel system in the intraradicular restoration of structurally compromised roots. *Quintessence Int* 1996 ; **27:** 483-491.

IN BRIEF

- Clarification of some of the terminology and concepts relating to occlusion as it is used in everyday practice, making clear why these concepts matter
- Undertaking a simple pre-operative examination of the occlusion as a matter of routine
- Helping clinicians identify cases where articulated study casts will help plan treatment and design restorations
- Advice is provided about selecting an appropriate articulator and taking appropriate records at the treatment stage.

Crowns and other extra-coronal restorations: Occlusal considerations and articulator selection

J. G. Steele[1] F. S. A. Nohl[2] and R. W. Wassell[3]

For many dentists, occlusion carries an air of mystique. It even seems sometimes that a perverse pleasure is derived in making the whole subject more complicated than it really is. As a clinician, you need to be able to decide what you expect from your proposed restoration, and to identify situations where you may need to alter the existing occlusal scheme. At a fundamental level, you also need to provide the laboratory with appropriate clinical records to ensure that when you fit them, adjustments to the expensively prepared restorations are minimal. This requires a sound understanding of the basics.

[1,3]Senior Lecturer in Restorative Dentistry, Department of Restorative Dentistry, The Dental School, Framlington Place, Newcastle upon Tyne NE2 4BW
[2]Consultant in Restorative Dentistry, The Dental Hospital, Framlington Place, Newcastle upon Tyne NE2 4AZ
*Correspondence to: J. G. Steele
E-mail: jimmy.steele@ncl.ac.uk

This fifth article in the series will try to present important occlusal concepts in a way which relates directly to the provision of successful crowns. It is not a comprehensive guide to occlusion, or a manual of techniques for extensive fixed prosthodontics. There are several useful books and articles dedicated to the subject and some of these are specifically referenced (if a technique is particularly well described) or are listed in the further reading section. However, we hope that this article should allow you to avoid most of the problems associated with the provision of crowns. Occasionally some pre-operative occlusal adjustment is needed. Our experience is that this is best taught 'hands on' and we would recommend attending an appropriate course before attempting more complex adjustments.

BASIC CONSIDERATIONS – WHAT MATTERS?

One of the essential starting points with occlusion is to make sure that the terminology is clear. There are any number of occlusal terms, many of which overlap. There are only a few that really matter and these need to be understood if what is to follow is to make any sense.

The intercuspal position (ICP or IP)

Synonyms: centric occlusion (CO), maximum intercuspation

What is it?

Most dentate patients, when asked simply to 'bite together on your back teeth', close immediately into a comfortable, reproducible "closed" position where the maximum number of tooth contacts occur. This is the intercuspal position (ICP). Travel into this position is partly guided by the shape of teeth and partly by conditioned neuromuscular co-ordination.[1] ICP is the most 'closed' position of the jaws.

Why does this matter?

ICP is usually the position in which vertical occlusal forces are most effectively borne by the periodontium with teeth likely to be loaded axially, which helps to stabilise their position. Indeed it is the end point of the chewing cycle where maximum force is exerted. In everyday practice this is the position of the jaws in which restorations are made.

Guidance (from the teeth)

What is it?

When a patient moves their mandible from side to side so that the teeth in opposing jaws slide over each other, the path taken is determined partly by the shapes of the teeth which make contact, as well as by the anatomical constraints of the temporomandibular joints (TMJs) and masticatory neuromuscular function. Each has a bearing on the other, and, for want of a better term, they should work in *harmony*. In these circumstances the teeth provide *guidance* for the movement of the mandible. The shape and form of the temporomandibular joints also guide the movement of the mandible (sometimes called posterior guidance). Guidance teeth can be any teeth, anterior or posterior.

When the patient slides the mandible out to one side, the side they move the mandible towards is called the *working side* (because it is usually the side on which they are about to

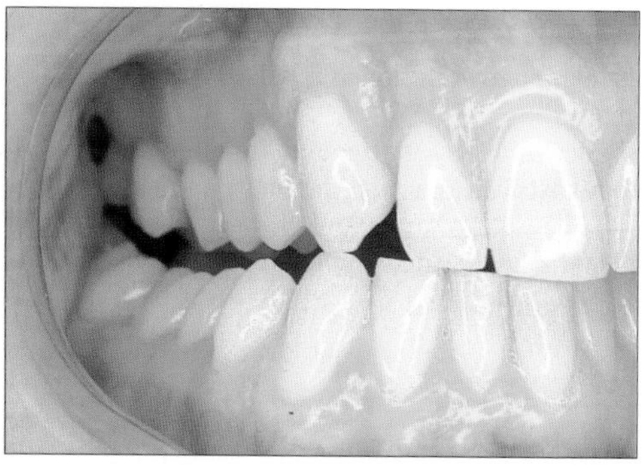

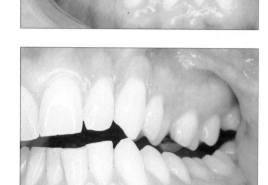

Fig. 1 Right canine guidance during right lateral excursion. Posterior teeth are discluded but contact remains between the lateral incisors

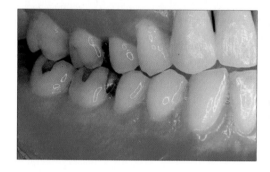

Fig. 2 Left canine guidance during left lateral excursion. Here the canines are the only teeth in contact

Fig. 3 Shared contact between many posterior teeth in right lateral excursion. Guidance is described as being group function

ture or decementation, particularly if these loads are heavy. Other manifestations of problems with guidance include:

- Fractured teeth or restorations
- Accelerated local wear
- Tooth migration
- Tooth mobility
- TMJ dysfunction

To avoid these it is important to identify which teeth provide guidance before you start tooth preparation. If the guidance is satisfactory, and the guidance tooth or teeth are strong enough to withstand the likely loading in the long term, it is usually best to try to re-establish the same guidance pattern in the new restoration. Techniques for doing this are described later in the article. Occasionally, you may feel that a tooth that you are about to crown is insufficiently robust to carry a guidance contact and the guidance is best moved onto other teeth. A specific example of this would be where a broken down guidance canine is restored with a post retained crown. There may be a risk of root fracture of the tooth in the longer term because of the heavy lateral forces. In a case like this, by taking a little care with the shape of both preparation and crown, guidance can often be transferred from the canine to the premolars, if they are in a better position to accept the heavy loads.

Other practical reasons for identifying guidance teeth include:

- The need to provide clearance from the opposing tooth during preparation, not just in ICP, but also along the guidance track. If you do not do this you can end up unwittingly transferring all the guidance forces on to your new crown.
- The need to select and prescribe an appropriate material to restore the guidance surface (metal is usually best if possible).

These aspects are discussed in detail later in the series.

The message is that getting guidance right is one of the most important aspects of crown provision; problems can, and will, occur unless guidance is correctly managed on teeth to be crowned.

chew). The other side, the side the mandible is moving away from, is called the *non-working side*. So for example, an excursion to the right (as may occur during chewing) will make the right side the working side and the left the non-working side, whilst during an excursion to the left the reverse will be true. During these excursions the upper and lower *guidance teeth* will be in contact and partly dictate the movement of the mandible. *Canine guidance* is where the upper and lower canines on the working side are the only teeth in contact during a lateral excursion, causing all of the posterior teeth to disclude (Figs 1 and 2). When several pairs of teeth, usually premolars or premolars and canines (and sometimes molars) on the working side share the contacts during excursions *group function* is said to take place (Fig. 3). Other patterns of guidance can take place, using almost any combination of teeth.

Incisors and canines usually provide protrusive guidance, when the mandible slides forward, but where there is only a limited overbite the posterior teeth may be involved.

Why does it matter?
Guidance teeth are repeatedly loaded non-axially (laterally) during excursions. As a result heavily restored or crowned teeth may be at risk of frac-

Interferences
What are they?
Interferences are any tooth-to-tooth contact(s), which hamper or hinder smooth guidance in excursions or closure into ICP. An interference on the side to which the mandible is moving is called a working side interference. An interference on the side from which the mandible is moving is called a non-working side interference (NWSI) or balancing side interference. There is a distinction to make between NWSIs and non-working side *contacts*: in the latter case, excursions are guided equally by working and non-working tooth contacts, akin to the *balanced articulation* often taught as an ideal complete denture occlusion. However, where

there is a NWSI it acts as a cross arch pivot, disrupting the smooth movement and separating guidance teeth on the working side (Fig. 4).

Why does it matter?

There has been much written about the significance or otherwise of interferences, particularly NWSIs, in relation to initiating parafunction and TMJ dysfunction. Warnings of the direst consequences to the stomatognathic system and beyond from NWSIs are frankly misleading though. Many people function perfectly happily with a mouthful of NWSIs. However, when contemplating crowns there are important implications. Most NWSIs are on molars so teeth or restorations directly involved are subject to high and often oblique occlusal forces with the consequent risk of fracture or uncementing.

As a general rule, it is best to remove interferences before tooth preparation if the interference is on a tooth which is to be prepared. This applies to all types of interference – working, non-working and protrusive. In practice it is best to do this at a separate appointment prior to tooth preparation. This will allow the patient time to adapt to a new pattern of excursive guidance, and you time to refine the guidance if necessary. The process of dealing with a non-working side interference prior to preparation is shown in Figure 4. If you do this, it is important to identify suitable teeth on the working side to take over the guidance once the interference has been eliminated. If there are no teeth to take over the guidance, it may be impossible to eliminate the NWSI. If you are in any doubt it would be best to seek advice before cutting the tooth.

Where interferences exist on teeth that are not themselves to be prepared, the need for adjustment may be less important. Many people have asymptomatic interferences and seem to be able to lead a normal existence and we certainly would not advocate the removal of all interferences as a public health measure.

One final point is that it is disturbingly easy to introduce new interferences when you place restorations, even where there were no interferences previously. If you check your preparations for adequate clearance, not only in ICP but in lateral and protrusive excursions as well, the chances of this occurring should be minimised. Obviously, there is the opportunity to remove minor interferences on the final restoration before cementation.

Retruded Contact Position (RCP)

Synonyms: centric relation (CR), centric relation contact position (CRCP), retruded axis position (RAP), terminal hinge position.

What is it?

This is the position of the mandible when the first contact between opposing teeth takes place, during closure on its hinge axis (or retruded arc of closure), that is with the condyles maximally seated in their fossae. This *condylar* position is one of health. Generally, as the mandible hinges

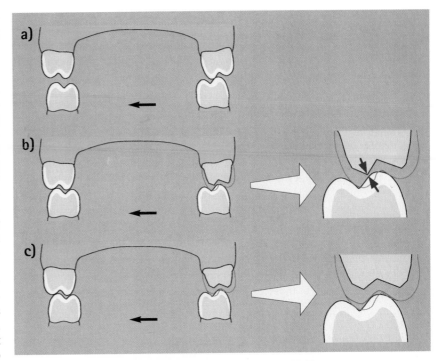

Fig. 4 A non-working side interference between the left first molars and the possible consequences of carrying out crown preparation without appreciating its presence (transverse section): a) During a right lateral excursion (see black arrow) the left first molars act as a cross-arch pivot lifting the teeth out of contact on the working side; b) The maxillary first molar has been prepared for a crown. Occlusal reduction has eliminated the pivot, allowing the teeth on the working side to contact during lateral excursion. However, clearance between the preparation and opposing teeth is now inadequate which may cause problems with the provisional restoration. Worse still, the definitive restoration may require gross adjustment resulting in its perforation; c) You can avoid these problems by removing the non-working side contact prior to tooth preparation (blue line represents tooth recontoured in this way)

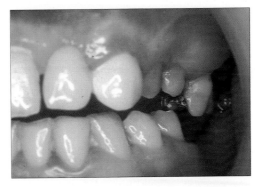

Fig. 5 A retruded contact between maxillary molar and mandibular premolar. Most retruded contacts cause no problems. This one resulted from over-eruption of the molar and the interference was associated with accelerated wear of the incisors

closed with the condyles in this position, there is a contact between a pair of teeth somewhere around the mouth (Fig. 5). The mandible will then close, from this retruded contact, down into ICP, usually sliding forward and laterally (Fig. 6). If you want to try to manipulate a patient's mandible into this position it is important that they are relaxed (Fig. 7), otherwise it can be very difficult and you will feel resistance to free movement of the mandible. For about 10% of people ICP will be the same as RCP[2] and in these cases if you hinge the mandible until the teeth are in contact they will go straight into ICP with no deflective contact.

Why does it matter?

There is no magic quality about RCP, but there are a number of reasons why RCP and the associated slide into ICP may be relevant when providing crowns. Box 1 contains a more detailed

BOX 1: RCP AND CROWNS

Most crowns and other extra-coronal restorations will be made to conform with the patient's ICP and usually a slide from RCP to ICP will be of no major relevance when providing crowns. In some circumstances additional management may be appropriate. The following are the situations where adjusting the contact in RCP is likely to be most important:

1. As a general rule, when RCP involves a tooth you are about to prepare it is often best to remove the deflective contact at an appointment before you start tooth preparation.
2. When re-organising the occlusion at a new vertical dimension you really have no option but to construct the new occlusion, if not at RCP itself , certainly around centric relation (with the condyles in the hinge axis). This represents the only reproducible starting point.
3. If you need space but you wish to avoid increasing the vertical dimension, there may be the scope to 'distalise' the mandible to create space lingually for anterior crowns (only possible where there is a bodily translation between RCP and ICP).
4. If you are about to restore anterior teeth and the RCP contact results in a strong anterior thrust against the teeth to be prepared.

Although we would usually advise removal of a deflective RCP interference before preparation if it is on a tooth you are about to prepare for a crown, many dentists do no not carry out any such adjustment and no problems result. This is probably because cutting the crown preparation effectively removes the contact. By removing it before preparation though you can ensure sufficient removal of tissue to allow space for the crown without re-introducing it in an uncontrolled way when the restoration is made. The principles involved are the same as those for removing non-working side interferences (see Fig. 4).

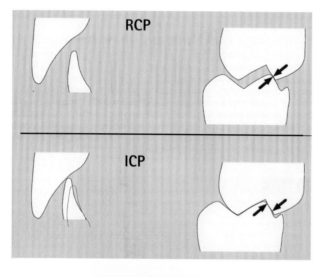

Fig. 6 The slide from retruded contact position (RCP) to the intercuspal position (ICP). Here, in RCP the molars make first contact as shown by the arrows. The magnitude and direction of the slide can be estimated at both the molar and incisor regions

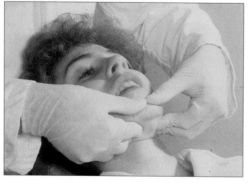

Fig. 7 One method of manipulating the mandible of a relaxed patient into the hinge axis position. This technique is called bimanual manipulation and is designed to seat the condyles fully in their fossae with the disks interposed

analysis of the situations where it may be a problem. In many, but not all cases, managing RCP is of less significance than managing guidance effectively, but there are times when adjustments need to be made and, clearly, it is always better to identify potential problems than blindly to hope for the best. To this end it is always worth examining RCP pre-operatively so that you at least know where it is. On the very few occasions where it is likely to be a major factor affecting your restorative procedure, casts mounted in RCP (or in the hinge axis just before

the teeth actually contact) on a semi-adjustable articulator will facilitate occlusal examination and allow trial adjustments.

Establishing and recording RCP, and particularly re-organising the occlusion, are often difficult and we would refer you to Further Reading below if you wish to follow these subjects up in more detail.

PRACTICAL ASPECTS OF OCCLUSION: RECORDS FOR PLANNING CROWNS

Records for planning crowns: The occlusal examination

Before providing crowns it really is mandatory to undertake some sort of an occlusal examination. The following observations take moments to gather and are worth the effort:

- Check ICP (for reproducibility and contacts on the teeth to be restored)
- Check RCP (to establish whether there is any deflective contact or slide which you ought to know about). For technique see Reference 3.
- Check the relationship of the teeth in lateral and protrusive excursions (to determine whether your crowns will be involved in guidance or if you need to consider removing an interference).

A more detailed and lengthy examination, where all of the contacts are marked using good quality ultra thin articulating tape (Fig. 8) is sometimes indicated, particularly where there has been a history of temporomandibular dysfunction or where there is a specific occlusal problem which you need to address. The various components, which may be included in a full occlusal examination, are given in Box 2.

Records for planning crowns: hand–held study casts

Hand-held casts can be a very useful aid to examination and treatment planning. To glean maximum information from them they need to be made from good quality impressions, which have been handled and poured correctly. We will return to this important but underrated subject later (see below: 'Opposing Casts').

Hand-held study casts enable:

- A judgement to be made regarding the ease of obtaining a stable ICP. This helps to determine whether or not an interocclusal record is required for the working casts upon which the restoration(s) will be made.
- An unimpeded view of ICP. It is possible to view aspects such as the lingual, which it would not be possible to see at the chairside.
- Careful evaluation of clinical crown height and the availability of inter-occlusal space for restorative material. These two factors can help make the decision on how to facilitate the restoration of short teeth (see Part 3 'Pre-operative assessment' in this series).

However tempting it may be to assume otherwise, hand-held casts provide no information about excursive tooth contacts or RCP, beyond the distribution of wear facets.

Records for planning crowns: Articulated study casts

Accurate casts of the dental arches mounted in a semi adjustable articulator are the most important tools of the trade when constructing artificial crowns. The need for an articulator and the positions in which you mount the casts depend on what you need to do (see Box 3). Articulators are surrounded by an aura of mystery, but at the end of the day they are a tool to help give your patient a successful restoration and to help you to save time, money and hassle. The quality of the final result is much less dependent on the articulator you use than it is on the care you exercise to make and mount the casts that you put in it.

There is little merit in examining study casts for planning purposes on a simple hinge or other 'non-anatomical' articulator because the ability to replicate physiological movements will be, at best, crude, and at worst, wholly misleading. A non-anatomical articulator will allow casts to be put into a reproducible ICP, which may be helpful if there are insufficient contacts to make hand-held casts stable, but that is the limit of what a simple hinge articulator can do.

BOX 2: COMPONENTS OF AN OCCLUSAL EXAMINATION

A full occlusal examination including all of the components below is rarely indicated, but different components may be required at different times. Visual assessments of ICP, RCP and guidance teeth are always indicated where you are planning crowns. The following may also be useful:

1. Examining for signs of temporomandibular dysfunction:
   - Palpation of muscles of mastication for tenderness.
   - Palpation of the temporomandibular joints and detailed assessment of any clicks or deviations in mandibular movement.
   - Assessment of the range of mandibular movement.

2. Checking for facets, fremitus, mobility and drifting (particularly where there are problems with individual teeth).

3. Marking up of the dry teeth in different coloured tapes (Fig. 8) to show contacts in all excursions using a high quality articulating tape (where there are issues affecting the entire occlusal scheme).

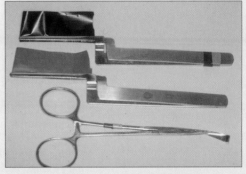

Fig. 8 Tools for examining occlusal contacts: foil shimstock held in forceps and high quality ultra-thin articulating tapes held in Millers forceps

---

BOX 3: WHEN TO USE A SEMI-ADJUSTABLE ARTICULATOR DURING THE MANUFACTURE OF CROWNS

1. If you wish to ensure appropriate guidance with your new restorations, particularly where multiple crowns are involved.

2. If you plan to increase the vertical dimension at all.

3. In any case where either you are going to remove so many of the occlusal contacts that ICP will effectively be lost and/or where you plan to make a new ICP based on RCP (sometimes known as a reorganised occlusion).

4. Where you plan to remove occlusal interferences (the study casts can enable a trial adjustment to be carried out).

5. When there is a need to provide an occlusal stabilisation appliance (occlusal splint), either before treatment to stabilise jaw position or after treatment to protect restorations from the effects of bruxism.

BOX 4: TAKING A GOOD OPPOSING IMPRESSION

1. Choose stock impression trays with adequate rigidity which, perhaps in combination with an adhesive, have sufficient retentive features to hold set alginate securely.

2. If the restoration is on a very posterior tooth you may need to extend the tray with a rigid material (green stick or compo but not carding wax) to ensure that the alginate is supported in important posterior areas.

3. Make sure adhesive has been air dried in the tray before loading alginate. Lots of wet adhesive acts as a lubricant not an adhesive, and if the alginate pulls away from the tray you are left with an enormous but not very obvious distortion in the final cast.

4. Dry the teeth with gauze or cotton wool to remove saliva, which aids tremendously in recording occlusal detail and producing of a smooth, hard cast surface. It can be done as the alginate is being mixed.

5. Smear a little alginate firmly onto the dry occlusal surfaces with your finger as the assistant finishes loading the tray.

After removal

6. Check to make sure the material has not pulled out of the tray (Fig. 9). If it has, retake it and do not assume it will be all right or be tempted to press dislodged material back into place; you will pay in the time spent adjusting the final crown.

7. Cut off the heels of the impression flush with the tray if you do not need them, they are prone to distort when you lay the impression down on the bench or even when it is loaded with wet stone. This takes seconds.

8. If you get the chance, check the casts, if not, ask the technician to do this and to flick off any air bubbles on critical surfaces (Fig. 10).

9. In really critical cases, consider using silicone to obtain a very accurate opposing cast especially if there is to be a delay before pouring up.

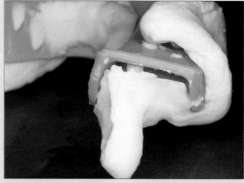

Fig. 9 Impression material has been pulled away from the tray on withdrawal from the mouth.
This will equate to at least a 1mm occlusal error

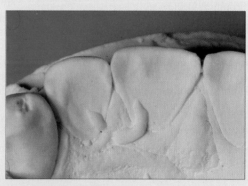

Fig. 10 Large stone blebs on the palatal surfaces of upper anterior teeth as a result of air bubbles in the impression

The combination of a facebow record (which locates the approximate position of the condylar hinge axis in relation to the upper arch) and a jaw relation record (which then locates the lower cast to the upper), enables movements of casts articulated on a semi-adjustable articulator to be reasonably anatomical. You can simulate the movements of the teeth in lateral and protrusive excursions, and around the hinge axis and be confident that what you see is close to what is really happening in the mouth. However, whilst the instrument is key, the quality of the casts and the care with which they are mounted are just as critical. There is no room for carelessness at this stage, wrongly articulated casts are probably worse than no casts at all as they may result in false assumptions about treatment. Similarly, inaccuracies with the original impressions can result in profound errors and the use of an accurate and stable impression material (such as addition cured silicone) may be appropriate in cases where a detailed occlusal analysis is necessary. Details of how to record a facebow record and a retruded hinge axis inter-occlusal record can be found in References 3 and 4. Some simple tips on accurate impression recording can be found in Box 4.

Although you can see and reproduce movements with carefully articulated casts, you may often want to go on to the next stage and prepare a diagnostic wax up.

Records for planning crowns: the diagnostic wax-up

In addition to its uses in planning changes in appearance (see Aesthetic Control – the sixth article in this series), a diagnostic wax-up can be an absolutely invaluable technique where you are changing the occluding surfaces of several teeth with crowns or resin bonded restorations and allows you to plan the following:

- The new static occlusal contacts (in ICP) and the shape of the guidance teeth
- The impact that the modified occlusion has on appearance
- The best options for creating interocclusal space for restoration(s) or optimising crown height by periodontal surgery (see Part 3: 'Pre–operative Assessment' in this series).

You can also use the completed wax-up as a template to determine the form of temporary and final restorations.

PRACTICAL ASPECTS OF OCCLUSION: RECORDS FOR MAKING CROWNS

When the diagnosis stage has been completed, the crowns or restorations still need to be made, and various records are essential at this stage too. This section discusses the choice of articulator and the need to obtain accurate occlusal records, including the simplest things such as opposing impressions, which are a frequent source of error. Finally, it introduces ways of controlling guidance on front teeth.

The articulator

When manufacturing the final crowns, in the interests of simplicity and cost it would seem sensible to use the simplest cast relating device that will not compromise the final restoration.[5] Small numbers of restorations, which are not involved in excursive contacts, can very reasonably be made on a non-adjustable articulator and then any adjustments made in the mouth before final cementation. However, crowns involved in excursions benefit from the use of an articulator with anatomical dimensions so that the excursive movements can be made and the shape of the crown adjusted in the lab with reasonable accuracy, saving chairside time. This becomes particularly important, and cost effective, when several restorations are being created at the same time. Highly sophisticated semi-adjustable and fully adjustable articulators are available for this purpose, but the majority of cases can be managed quite satisfactorily using a less sophisticated, fixed average value articulator in combination with a facebow.

It may not be possible to check occlusion on adhesive restorations prior to cementation, either because the act of checking may damage porcelain, which is delicate until cemented, or because they will not stay in place during excursions. In these cases, controlling the role of the restorations in guidance can be critical to their long-term survival. A semi-adjustable articulator can be invaluable in situations such as these because it allows the technician to secure restorations onto the working cast and do the critical adjustments in the lab so that all you need to do is cement them with little or no adjustment afterwards.

Opposing casts

In any discussion about articulators, it is disturbingly easy to forget the importance of an accurate cast to oppose the working cast. The opposing impression is often the last thing we do and, after a long session preparing teeth, making temporaries and taking impressions it tends to be a bit of an afterthought. However, a poor opposing impression is very easy indeed to achieve and yet can cost a great deal of precious time subsequently. A cast made with a distorted impression or a porous impression resulting in plaster blebs on occlusal surfaces will not fit comfortably into ICP. If such a cast is used in the lab it can result in a crown which looks perfectly good on the cast but which may be very high in the ICP and which can take a great deal of time to get right prior to fit. It is easy to record bad opposing impressions, but good ones are just as easy. Attention to the few steps listed in Box 4 takes, literally, no extra time but can save a lot of heartache. In an ideal world every opposing impression would be recorded in a dimensionally accurate and stable material such as an addition cured silicone, but

this is probably not economically realistic. Box 4 describes the use of alginate for an opposing impression. In cases involving multiple restorations though, a very stable and accurate material may be cost effective in the long term.

Interocclusal records (IOR)

Once you have your working impression and opposing impression you then need to decide whether you need to provide additional information to the lab to allow them to mount the casts; an inter-occlusal record (IOR). There is a common perception that providing an intercuspal record (such as a wax or silicone 'bite') will improve the accuracy of mounted casts. The truth is that in many cases it does precisely the opposite.[6]

For a patient with a stable intercuspal position, the loss of interocclusal contact created by preparation of a tooth for a single unit restoration, is unlikely to detract from the ease with which working and opposing casts can be located in ICP. In this circumstance, placing a layer of wax or silicone between the casts to help to locate them can often result in them failing to seat into ICP at all, and there is a very serious risk of the record introducing inaccuracies, rather than acting as the 'insurance policy' you intended. It is worth taking the opportunity of examining the ease with which any study casts can be located by hand before deciding whether an IOR is needed. Often (perhaps even usually) you are better with nothing at all.

Sometimes an IOR is required to stabilise casts, particularly where the teeth that are prepared are key support teeth in an arch. The choice of materials is generally between hard wax alone, hard wax (as a carrier) used with zinc oxide/eugenol, silicone elastomers and acrylic resins. The fundamental requirement is to obtain enough detail in a dimensionally stable recording material to enable casts to be confidently located in the laboratory whilst not recording so much detail that it stops the casts seating. Occlusal fissure patterns reproduced accurately in the IOR may well not be reproduced to the same extent in the cast, preventing full seating of the casts in the record. Furthermore, an IOR which contacts soft tissues in the mouth and causes their displacement (which is obviously not reproduced in the stone cast) will result in an IOR which will not seat accurately (Figs 11 and 12). In order to meet the requirements for success, an IOR should:

1. Record the tips of cusps or preparations
   BUT
2. Avoid capturing fissure patterns as much as possible
   AND
3. Avoid any soft tissue contact

The key to a successful record is not so much the type of material used, but how it is used. The smaller the amount you use, the less it is likely to cause a problem. A small, trimmed record, restricted to the area of the preps themselves,

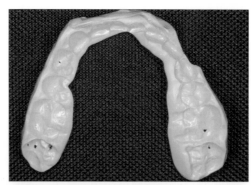

Fig. 11 A very accurate full arch occlusal record in a silicone material. The excessive detail may well hinder seating on a stone cast. See Fig. 12

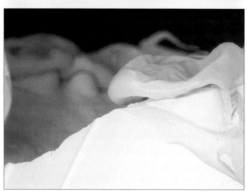

Fig. 12 The combination of a very detailed silicone occlusal record and less detailed stone cast, particularly of the occlusal fissures, has meant that the record will not seat. There were sufficient tooth contacts in the intercuspal position not to need an interocclusal record for this case!

with all interproximal tags and undercuts removed is the ideal. It is usually necessary to trim the record to achieve these requirements and silicone materials trim very easily with a scalpel (Fig. 13). One final consideration is that stone casts and dies can easily be abraded by IORs especially those made of acrylic resin and special care is required in the laboratory when these materials are used in combination.

Whether or not you have used an interocclusal record, you can easily verify the accuracy of mounted casts in the ICP using foil shimstock. When held tightly together the cast should hold the shim between the same teeth as they do in the mouth.

Copying tooth guidance

When a restoration is being provided which includes a guiding surface for mandibular excursions (lateral, protrusive or anything in between), the technician needs to know what form the contacting surface is to take. Failure to appreciate this risks introducing excursive contacts that are not in harmony with the other guidance teeth, the condylar movements and musculature. This is discussed fully earlier in the article, but common manifestations of disharmony include:

- Decementing and fractured crowns
- Tooth mobility
- Tooth migration
- TMJ dysfunction

Because they are intimately involved in speech formation, getting guidance wrong on the palatal surfaces of upper anterior teeth may also come to light as phonetic problems.

The guidance of a new restoration can often be made simply to fit in with that provided by adjacent teeth (for example in group function). In

this case the new functional surface is relatively straightforward to achieve on a semi-adjustable articulator or even at the chairside. However, if several teeth are to be prepared there may be no existing guiding surfaces left intact after preparation, so all clues to guidance are lost (Fig. 14). Where satisfactory guidance is present before you start, there are several ways of copying it before you prepare the teeth. A commonly used technique is to use a putty matrix made on a cast of the tooth surfaces to be copied, but this technique will often not provide the tight control over tooth shape which is required. The two most effective methods to address this problem necessitate the use of a facebow and semi-adjustable articulator to allow anatomical movements in excursions. They are:

1. *The 'crown about' method:* Alternate teeth are restored, thus maintaining the shapes of functional surfaces, which continue to provide guidance for the articulated casts. This technique is well described in Reference 7.
2. *The custom incisal guide table:* This is another way of copying satisfactory anterior guidance from teeth or trial restorations that provide crucial excursive contacts. Unlike the previous method, it enables guidance to be copied for just one restoration. It involves moving study casts (on a semi-adjustable articulator) through the full range of lateral and protrusive excursions with a mound of un-set acrylic on the guide table, so that the tip of the articulator guide pin shapes the acrylic dough

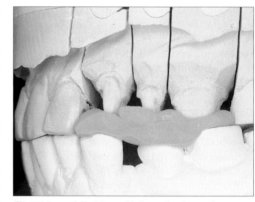

Fig. 13 A carefully trimmed interocclusal record restricted to the area of tooth preparation. The resulting crowns needed no adjustment

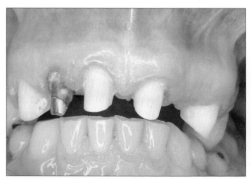

Fig. 14 Preparation of the teeth has resulted in loss of all guiding surfaces on the anterior teeth

into (once set) a permanent record of the movements of the mandible (Fig. 15). When the working casts are articulated the acrylic guide table guides the articulator through the same movements that were present in the study casts, and the palatal surfaces of the upper teeth can be shaped to conform precisely to this. This technique is described in detail, with illustrations, in Reference 4.

The extra effort involved in using these techniques is not enormous, and where several anterior teeth are to be crowned we would strongly recommend using one or other of them.

1. Okeson J P. *Management of temporomandibular disorders and occlusion.* 1998. 4th Edition. St Louis: Mosby, pp47-51.
2. Posselt U. Studies in the mobility of the human mandible. *Acta Odontol Scand* 1952; **10** : 109.
3. Wise D. Occlusion and restorative dentistry for the general practitioner. Part 2- Examination of the occlusion and fabrication of study casts. *Br Dent J* 1982; **152:** 160-165.
4. Howat A P, Capp N J, Barrett N V J. A colour atlas of occlusion and malocclusion. 1991. London: Wolfe Publishing, pp137-139.
5. Loos L G. Clinical criteria used to select an articulator. *Compend Contin Educ Dent* 1993; **14:** 80-88.
6. Walls A W G, Wassell R W, Steele J G. A comparison of two methods for locating the intercuspal position (ICP) whilst mounting casts on an articulator. *J Oral Rehabil* 1991; **18:** 43-48.
7. Wise D. Occlusion and restorative dentistry for the general practitioner. Part 9 – Restoration of anterior teeth. *Br Dent J* 1982; **152:** 407-413.

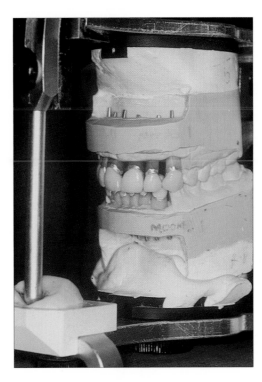

Fig. 15 A custom acrylic guide table for use with a semi-adjustable articulator. This is an excellent method of copying tooth guidance into definitive restorations

Further reading

1. Wise M. Occlusion and restorative dentistry for the general practitioner. Series of ten articles published in the Br Dent J 1982; **152**: 117; **152**: 160; **152**: 197; **152**: 235; **152**: 277; **152**: 316; **152**: 347; **152**: 381; **152**: 407; **153**: 13.
2. Howat A P, Capp N J, Barrett N V J. A colour atlas of occlusion and malocclusion. 1991. London: Wolfe Publishing.
3. Shillingburg H T Jr, Hobo S, Whitset L D, Jacobi R, Brackett S E. Fundamentals of fixed prosthodontics. 3rd ed. 1997. London: Quintessence Publishing Co.

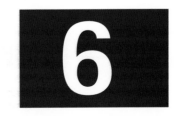

IN BRIEF

- Identification and definition of the patient's aesthetic problem
- Consideration of the balance between aesthetics and tooth destruction for conventional and adhesive restorations
- An awareness of the aesthetic limitations of restorations and an attempt to ensure that the patient's expectations are realistic
- Incorporation of procedures leading to better aesthetics at each clinical stage
- Confidence in determining shade and communicating effectively with the laboratory

Crowns and other extra-coronal restorations: Aesthetic control

F. S. A. Nohl[1] J. G. Steele[2] and R. W. Wassell[3]

A pleasing dental appearance is the subjective appreciation of the shade, shape and arrangement of the teeth and their relationship to the gingiva, lips and facial features. Achieving such a pleasing appearance in our patients is not always easy but is critical, not least because our work is effectively on display and this has implications for patients' perceptions of our practice. To be successful, thorough assessment, careful planning and precise clinical execution is required. Every bit as important though, is good communication, both with the dental laboratory and particularly with the patient. In few areas of dentistry can effective communication be as critical as it is here.

[1]Consultant in Restorative Dentistry, The Dental Hospital, Framlington Place, Newcastle upon Tyne NE2 4AZ
[2,3]Senior Lecturer in Restorative Dentistry, Department of Restorative Dentistry, The Dental School, Framlington Place, Newcastle upon Tyne NE2 4BW
*Correspondence to: F. S. A. Nohl
E-mail: f.s.a.nohl@newcastle.ac.uk

Retention of natural teeth into old age is now commonplace and whilst usually desirable, it has brought with it considerable additional problems. Making well-aligned white teeth in a complete denture is usually straightforward, but matching a single crown or veneer to a group of natural incisors is a different matter altogether. This problem is illustrated by data from the 1988 survey of adult dental health in the United Kingdom[1] which showed that having just one or two crowns was more likely to be associated with dissatisfaction with the appearance than having none or many.

In each case, planning tooth preparation involves the dentist in a cost:benefit analysis, where the cost of improved aesthetics is judged in terms of removal of tooth tissue and in the potential for damage to the pulp and periodontium. However the benefit of stunning porcelain work is easiest to achieve where a thick layer of material can be used to develop the optimum optical properties, but this usually requires more tooth tissue to be removed. This is a theme which runs right through all aesthetic considerations and should underpin what follows. This concept does not sit comfortably with a dogmatic approach with hard and fast rules about the dimensions of a preparation. The clinician will choose to alter the cost:benefit balance in different ways in different cases. The choice might be made to sacrifice aesthetics for long-term health, or to take a risk with long-term pulp health to maximise aesthetics; for example with a heavily prepared ceramo-metal restoration.

Aesthetic improvements are most important for anterior teeth and may often be the sole reason for providing the restoration. The type of materials used clearly have an important bearing on both the appearance and the amount of preparation and are an important part of the aesthetic cost:benefit equation. Table 1 lists the aesthetic restorations commonly available. Whilst they are much less destructive of tooth tissue than traditional ceramo-metal crowns, adhesive restorations such as the porcelain laminate veneer and dentine bonded crown do have limitations: specifically the problem of masking the colour of darkly stained teeth, problems of temporisation and the inability to cement restorations provisionally. Veneers are covered in detail in a separate article in this series (Part 12). Furthermore whilst there have been significant improvements in indirect composite technology

Table 1 Laboratory made aesthetic restorations

- All porcelain

  Conventional porcelain jacket crown

  High strength porcelain jacket crown

  Full coverage porcelain veneer (dentine bonded crown)

  Porcelain labial veneer

  Porcelain onlay

- All composite

  Crown

  Veneer

  Onlay

- Ceramo-metal crown
- Composite bonded to metal crown
- Partial coverage metal crown

Table 2 Factors contributing to dental aesthetics

Dental	Mucogingival	Facial	General
• Shade	• Margin level	• Lip levels at rest	• Age
• Contour	• Margin pattern	• Lip levels in function	• Occupation
• Texture	• Shape of papillae	• Centre line	• Gender
• Shape	• Colour		• Personality
• Position	• Thickness		
• Arrangement			
• Interproximal contacts			
• Incisal embrasures			
• Gingival embrasures			
• Incisal level			
• Posterior occlusal level			

there is as yet little clinical evidence of their stability and longevity.

The key decisions are similar for anterior or posterior teeth, but there is usually less room for aesthetic compromise at the front of the mouth. On posterior teeth it may be feasible to sacrifice optimum aesthetics by restricting the use of porcelain only to the most visible sites and consequently cutting a less damaging preparation. For example on a short tooth, creating space for occlusal porcelain and metal rather than for metal alone could make the difference between success and failure of retention. Furthermore, tooth preparation carries with it the risk of pulp damage.[2]

A conservative approach would equate not only to less pulp morbidity, but more tooth remaining should the need arise to remake the restoration. On a posterior tooth it may also be possible to use a three quarter crown, which leaves the bulk of the buccal surface intact. Once again, whatever the materials chosen, it is important that the patient fully understands the advantages and limitations of the restorative solution. This article aims to address all of these

issues. The field of dental aesthetics is highly subjective and, as a result, difficult to research. The advice we offer and the recommendations we give are necessarily based more on experience than scientific analysis.

IDENTIFYING THE PROBLEM

The first and fundamental key to obtaining a successful aesthetic result is to establish the precise nature of the patient's demands, at the outset of treatment. What is perceived as 'natural' or pleasing to the dentist or technician may be much too 'natural', and far from pleasing for the patient. This may sound obvious, but without a detailed assessment it is easy to fail to make a precise diagnosis of the patient's desires, and so end up treating something which is not a problem for the patient, or creating technically beautiful restorations which the patient perceives to be aesthetically unsatisfactory, with all the angst and cost that this implies.

Table 2 shows the many factors, which must be considered in defining the patient's aesthetic problem. On the basis of a thorough assessment, the dentist must decide whether:

- The patient's expectations are realistic
- The proposed treatment options are in the patient's best interests
- The dentist, with the support of the laboratory, has the skill to carry out the treatment.

One of the greatest challenges for dentists providing crowns and veneers is the need to match expectations to what is technically and aesthetically achievable.

Matching expectations with reality

Most patients appreciate a full and frank discussion about what is achievable. Time spent at this stage can save a lot of heartache and expense later on. There are reversible means of helping patients understand the scope and possible consequences of treatment:

- Wax mock-ups (diagnostic wax-ups) on stone casts can be very useful for demonstrating treatment options and act as blue-prints for carrying out clinical and laboratory work (Figs 1 and 2). Some dentists prefer these models to be created in tooth-coloured wax whilst others express concern that patients may not fully appreciate that these models are to assess shape not colour and for this reason deliberately use non tooth-coloured wax.
- Composite resin can be used on teeth in its uncured state to indicate the potential for shade and additive shape changes to natural teeth (Figs 3 to 5).
- When viewed against the darkness of the mouth, black, water-soluble ink can give a rough idea of the effect of subtractive shape changes such as shortening overerupted lower incisors (Fig. 4).
- Computer software, which can manipulate photographic images, is becoming commonplace in the dental surgery and can be useful in discussions of treatment options. However,

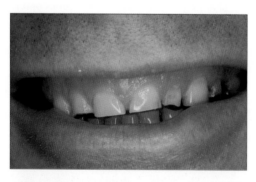

Fig. 1 Short anterior teeth causing an aesthetic problem

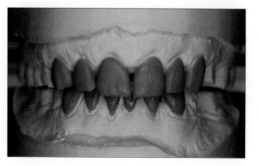

Fig. 2 Diagnostic wax-up of Case in figure 1

it is probably fair to say that it is much more difficult to provide restorations exactly as created on a screen than to use a wax model as a guide, especially if the patient has been given a colour enhanced print of the expected outcome! Unlike the techniques described above, computer manipulation of images has no physical limits and may as a result create unrealistic expectations.

- Photographs of previous cases may help patients to understand both the possibilities and the limitations. Restricting these to the ones with the best results may be a mistake. Where there are clearly going to be aesthetic limitations, it is probably best to illustrate them with realistic examples. The patient may be more likely to agree to treatment if they can picture the outcome, rather than imagine it from a verbal description.

- Provisional restorations can allow the subtle relationship between the shape and form of the teeth and the soft tissues and facial features to be evaluated and decided before the final restoration is constructed. They can also ensure that tooth preparation for restorative material is adequate (by establishing the desired shape and form and then measuring the thickness of temporaries with callipers).

Unrealistic expectations

Some patients may demand changes in appearance which are objectively difficult to appreciate and still more difficult to realise. In most cases this is simply a problem of communication, but unrealistic expectations and a history of multiple previous treatments addressing appearance may be a warning of a patient with Body Dysmorphic Disorder (BDD) or Dysmorphophobia[3]: a preoccupation with a defect in appearance which is either imagined or excessive in relation to a minor defect and which causes significant distress in social, occupational and other areas of life. BDD is probably rare but is an extraordinarily difficult problem to deal with. It is unlikely that demands to change appearance will be satisfied for this group of patients. A second opinion is a perfectly acceptable course of action if in doubt.

FINAL PLANNING AND CLINICAL PROCEDURES

Having decided on the restoration type, it remains to finalise margin features and carry out the clinical stages, ultimately leading to cementation.

Supra or sub-gingival: where should the crown margin go?

Factors identified in the assessment should help to determine the location of crown margins. Where the margins are not visible, there are good biological arguments for placing all margins supra-gingivally.[4] These sites would include all margins on molars, lingual and interproximal sites, and buccal aspects of

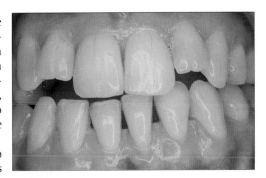

Fig. 3 Case requiring changes in upper lateral incisor length and levelling of lower incisal plane

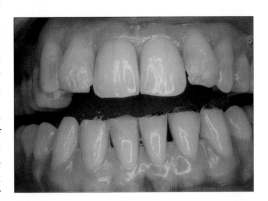

Fig. 4 Trial alterations to case in figure 3: uncured composite added to upper incisal edges and water-soluble ink to lower left incisors and canine

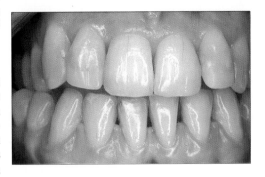

Fig. 5 Final restoration of upper lateral incisor edges of case in figure 3 (directly applied composite resin used in this instance)

anteriors and premolars where functional lip positions obscure the gingival margin. Not only will this facilitate finishing and maintenance but should also favour periodontal health. The appearance of a supragingival margin can be optimised by ensuring that the finish line is in harmony with the level of the gingival margin.

Where exposed crown margins are likely to create an aesthetic problem, margin placement up to 1 mm into the gingival sulcus can be acceptable.[5] However, great caution should be exercised as gingival margins are at risk of recession, particularly when there are prominent roots, thin gingival tissues or in the presence of periodontitis. Though periodontal attachment loss occurs to a greater or lesser degree through life,[6] trauma during clinical stages and poorly fitting temporary and final restorations will increase the risk of gingival inflammation and subsequent recession. The need to optimise retention by increasing preparation length may be better addressed by removing periodontal attachment surgically ('crown lengthening'), than by making the margin encroach deeply into the gingival sulcus and attachment apparatus with the risk of inflammation.

A guide to crowns

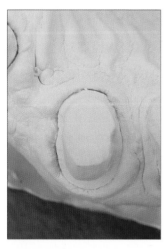

Fig. 6 Die with reduction to match veneering material(s): the larger buccal axial reduction is needed to accommodate metal and porcelain, the smaller palatal reduction is for metal alone

Shoulder or chamfer: what should the preparation finish line be like?

There is a forceful argument that where possible, ceramo-metal crowns should have metal margins because this produces the most predictable marginal seal[7] but as discussed earlier in this series (Part 2 'Materials Considerations'), this is a contentious issue. However by avoiding the metal collar, a porcelain butt fit, created on a shoulder finish line, will generally allow for better aesthetics in critical areas. A restoration whose margin is in porcelain may allow light to pass into porcelain from the gingival aspect as it does into intact teeth contributing to a lifelike appearance.[8]

How much metal: where should the porcelain-metal junction on ceramo-metal crowns be?

There is no biological or technical benefit in using porcelain at sites that are not visible. Consideration given to the precise location of porcelain-metal junctions for ceramo-metal crowns at the planning stage gives the potential to optimise conservation of tooth structure yet still maintain satisfactory aesthetics. Volume to volume, the extent of reduction for metal alone is substantially less than for metal and porcelain: different depths of tooth reduction can be used at different sites depending on the covering material(s). Tooth preparation then becomes an ordered technical exercise to satisfy the need for differential space attainment. It should be obvious to the technician examining the resulting die where to locate porcelain-metal junctions (Fig. 6). There are laboratory cost implications to provision of ceramo-metal crowns of this sort. It is necessary to wax a full contour restoration on the die, mark the porcelain-metal junction and then cut back space in the wax pattern for porcelain rather than simply to create a thin metal coping over the whole preparation which is covered by porcelain.

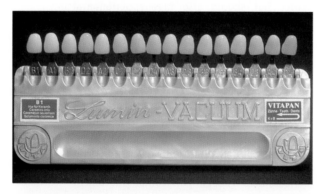

Fig. 7 Vita Lumin shade tabs with stained necks removed in order of decreasing value

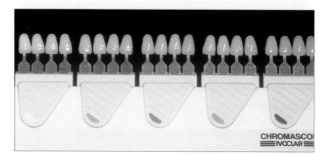

Fig. 8 Ivolcar Chromascop shade guide

Shade matching

Shade matching is something many of us find difficult and is often done last whereas in fact it should be done first! It is not an exact science, involving as it does a good deal of subjective judgement. Although an accurate reproduction of shade is an obvious goal, it cannot be divorced from consideration of shape, surface texture and special characteristics, which are described later. Teeth possess a range of optical features seemingly designed to make shade matching difficult! Teeth:

- Are non-uniform in colour
- May have complex visible internal and surface features
- Are semi-translucent
- Exhibit a degree of fluorescence
- Change shade and shape with age

In addition, a good shade match to porcelain in one light condition may be a poor one under different lighting: a phenomenon termed metamerism. Despite these obstacles, the best porcelain restorations go a long way to reproducing nature using a combination of skilful artistry and optical trickery. Before recording and prescribing shade it is useful to have a basic understanding of the science and dimensions of colour and texture so that shades can be interpreted and communicated precisely.

Dimensions of colour

Colour can be described in terms of three dimensions:

1. *Hue:* The name of the colour eg blue, red etc.
2. *Value:* An achromatic measure of the lightness or darkness of a particular colour such that high value refers to a shade which is light and low value to one which is dark. Two completely different colours can have exactly the same value. To help understand this, imagine the effect of black and white television on colours.
3. *Chroma:* The strength or saturation of a colour of particular hue. Imagine increasing the chroma of a small amount of colour pigment diluted in water by adding more of the same pigment.

Shade guides in common use (Figs 7 and 8) are not designed for a systematic assessment of the dimensions of colour and have been criticised for not including a broad enough range of shades. Two commonly used guides (Vita Lumin and Ivoclar Chromoscope) are composed of groups based essentially on hue (Vita Lumin: A= reddish brown, B = reddish yellow, C = grey shades, D = reddish grey, Ivoclar Chromascop: 1 series = cream, 2 series = orange, 3 series = light brown, 4 series = grey, 5 series = dark brown), with sub-classes of varying value and chroma. The Vitapan 3D Master system uses a simple but methodical approach to shade determination based on the three dimensions of colour. In common with previous work,[9] the

Vitapan 3D Master system emphasises value as the most important dimension in colour matching for porcelain restorations. Whichever guide is used, it is useful to understand colour terminology as it forms a language for communicating additional information about colour to the laboratory.

Surface texture
This quality describes surface contour both at a 'macro' level, such as developmental lobes and ridges, as well as fine surface detail such as perikymata. The lustre of a restoration describes the level of glaze produced in the porcelain oven or by various rotary instruments and polishing techniques. Lustre can effect value perception such that high lustre raises value. It is therefore an important feature to match and one which is often neglected. At the very least, terms such as high, medium or low lustre can be used on the prescription, and are more effective if they are linked to a standardised reference guide which can be used both in the surgery and in the dental laboratory. The technician can often get a good indication of other surface features from surrounding teeth.

Special characteristics
These include fracture lines, white spots and translucency. The best looking special characteristics are incorporated during incremental porcelain application. Surface stains can be used to produce some of these effects but are prone to wearing away with time.

Choosing and prescribing a shade
As well as factors inherent in teeth themselves, barriers to accurate shade matching often include inappropriate viewing conditions, shade guides that tend to be made from thick layers of high fusing porcelain and even colour blindness.[10] Against this background, it is perhaps not surprising that different dentists tend to match the same tooth differently from each other, and even from previous attempts to match the same tooth themselves.[11] Choosing a shade will benefit from adherence to a protocol based on sound reasoning. Table 3 gives a method for assessing shade and surface texture[12] which we think is highly appropriate and is easy to apply. Occasionally custom-made shade tabs with varying amounts of porcelains and a range of surface textures and special characteristics are helpful. Electronic optical devices have been produced to assist making an objective assessment of shade but their usefulness remains to be fully evaluated.

Tooth preparation
Achieving optimum aesthetics depends heavily on providing the technician with adequate space for the incremental application of porcelain (Fig. 9). The considerations have already been discussed above, but when it comes to the practicalities, the extent of tooth preparation is best visualised intra-orally by reference to a preparation guide. A small putty mould, made over the

Table 3 A scheme for shade determination	
1.	Determine shade at the start of an appointment before the risk of eye fatigue and tooth dehydration with resultant shade change (especially after use of rubber dam).
2.	Use either natural light (not direct sunlight) or a colour corrected artificial light source.
3.	Drape the patient with a neutral coloured cover if clothing is bright and have the patient remove brightly coloured makeup.
4.	Assess value by squinting. The reduced amount of light entering the eye may allow the retinal rods to better distinguish degrees of lightness and darkness. (Vita Lumin shade tabs set in order of value facilitates this [Fig. 7])
5.	Make rapid comparisons with shade tabs (no more than 5 seconds each viewing). Gazing at a soft blue colour between attempts is said to reduce blue fatigue, which can result in accentuation of yellow-orange sensitivity.
6.	Choose the dominant hue and chroma within the value range chosen. The canines have high chroma and may be a useful guide to assessing hue.
7.	Compare selected tabs under different conditions eg wet vs dry, different lip positions, artificial and natural light from different angles.
8.	Select a shade which is higher in value (lighter) if in doubt. Surface stains can reduce these dimensions but not easily increase them.
9.	Look carefully for colour characterisation such as stained imbrication lines, white spots, neck colouration, incisal edge translucency and halo effect (a thin opaque line sometimes seen within a translucent incisal). Shade tabs exactly representing the pure porcelains and stains available can be useful for this task. Simple diagrams are invaluable.
10.	Determine surface lustre.

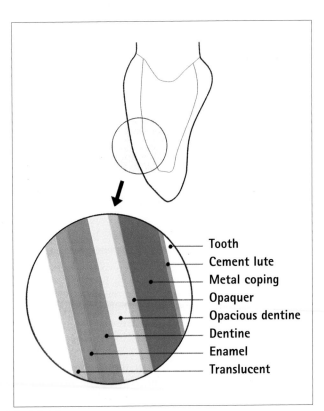

Tooth
Cement lute
Metal coping
Opaquer
Opacious dentine
Dentine
Enamel
Translucent

Fig. 9 Space required for metal coping and layers of porcelain for a ceramo–metal crown

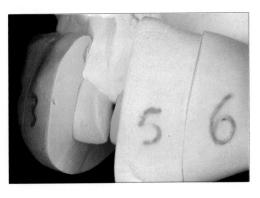

Fig. 10 Putty mould sectioned and numbered on a diagnostic wax-up

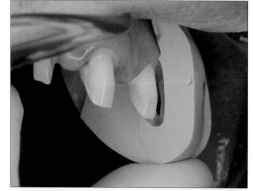

Fig. 11 Putty matrix in-situ to help visualise appropriate tooth reduction

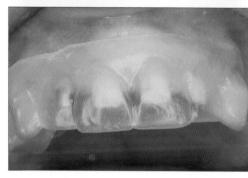

Fig. 12 Vacuum formed matrix in–situ

1. Todd J E, Lader D. *Adult Dental Health 1988: United Kingdom.* Office of Population Censuses and Surveys, 1991.
2. Saunders W P, Saunders E M. Prevalence of periradicular periodontitis associated with crowned teeth in an adult Scottish subpopulation. *Br Dent J* 1998; **185:** 137-140.
3. Cunningham S J, Bryant C J, Manisali M, Hunt H P, Feinman C. Dysmorphophobia: recent developments of interest to the maxillofacial surgeon. *Br J Oral and Maxillofac Surg* 1996; **34:** 368-374.
4. Valderhaug J, Birkeland J M. Periodontal conditions in patients 5 years following insertion of fixed prostheses. *J Oral Rehabil* 1976; **3:** 237-243.
5. Freilich M A, Niekrash C E, Katz R V, Simonsen R J. Periodontal effects of fixed partial denture retainer margins: configuration and location. *J Prosthet Dent* 1992; **67:** 184-190.

tooth before preparation, and then cut in cross-section is invaluable if the shape of the tooth is to be maintained. A putty mould (Figs 10 and 11) or vacuum formed matrix made from a diagnostic wax-up is required if the shape of the tooth is to be changed (Fig. 12). Depth cuts to guide tooth reduction may be a useful guide to ensure adequate reduction, but are not very helpful when shape changes are planned. Matrices are particularly helpful on the buccal surfaces of upper anterior teeth which are curved when viewed from the mesial or distal. There is a tendency to prepare the buccal surface in a single plane, ignoring the curvature (Fig. 13). The aesthetic result will either be a bulky crown (if the full thickness of porcelain is placed), or a crown where the contour is correct, but where the core porcelain is inadequately masked. To achieve a good aesthetic result the buccal surface preparation should follow the natural curvature of the tooth (see Fig. 11).

Clinical records
As well as the role of the facebow record in helping to make movements of casts on an articulator anatomical, it ensures that articulated working casts are orientated to the base of articulator in the same way that the patient's teeth are orientated with respect to the floor (if the patient's head is upright and the anatomical features used as reference points are normally related!). This helps the technician 'see' the restorations orientated as they would be when observing the patient. Very occasionally an ear-bow recording can give an erroneous interpretation of the relationship of the occlusal to the horizontal plane. This discrepancy occurs as a result of the patient's ears being at different levels and may need to be compensated for where multiple anterior crowns are prescribed.

Try-in and cementation
Where shade matching has been difficult for conventional crowns, there is merit in trial placement of moistened restorations before giving them their final surface finish. Surface stains and changes in surface form can be prescribed at this stage (Fig. 14). It should be remembered that surface stains might eventually be lost.

After glazing, a period of trial cementation leaves scope for a further period of assessment by both patient and dentist. If restorations are subsequently returned to the laboratory for adjustment, steps must be taken to dehydrate porcelain before firing to avoid the risk of fracture. Furthermore, temporarily cemented definitive crowns can be difficult to remove. Zinc oxide and eugenol-based cement must have its mechanical properties significantly reduced by adding a modifier as described later in this series (Part 11 'Try-in and cementation').

Pigmented luting agents allow subtle manipulation of shade for adhesive porcelain restorations. Some systems provide water-based trial cements to facilitate the choice of colour. Manufactures' instructions should be followed.

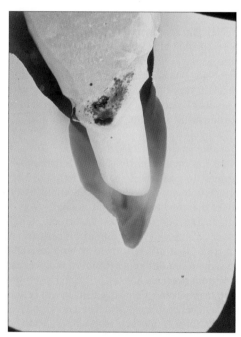

Fig. 13 Crown preparation with no second plane of reduction

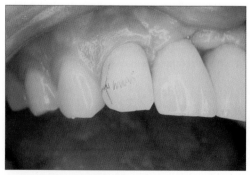

Fig. 14 Ceramo-metal crown at the pre-glaze stage. Along with written instructions, pencil marks help to indicate changes required

COMMUNICATION WITH THE LABORATORY

The dentist must accept ultimate responsibility for all aspects of completed laboratory work. On the face of it this might suggest that a totally prescriptive one-way communication is required. Not surprisingly such an attitude can lead to feelings of frustration and dissatisfaction to all concerned. It does not have to be like this! Trained technicians are highly skilled in a unique blend of art, craftsmanship and science (as can be appreciated very rapidly by any dentist attempting to wield wax or porcelain!). Better then to foster a team approach and central to a conflict free relationship is the establishment of dialogue and clearly defined roles for dentist and technician. To this end there is little to beat a personal visit to the laboratory and subsequently it is helpful to be available to speak to technicians and to share ideas. Certainly it is important at the very least to provide a clear written prescription which should include a diagram to enable regional variations in shade and special characteristics to be understood. Where there are difficulties in recording shade a wise dentist will involve the technician in the decision. Compliments as well as constructive criticism will help technicians evaluate their work, and anyone who takes pride in their work will appreciate the opportunity to see the final result of a job well done. It is probably fair to say that quality clinical work will be rewarded with higher quality restorations.

CONCLUSION

A complete understanding of a patient's aesthetic problems is the key to treatment planning. Only then can an attempt be made to match expectations with realities and to provide appropriate restorations. This process depends heavily on an understanding of the limitations of the techniques and materials available.

Manufacturers' details:
Ivoclar-Vivadent Ltd, Meridian South, Leicester LE3 2WY
VITA Zahnfabrik, H Rauter GmbH & Co KG, Postfach,
D-79704, Bad Säckingen, Germany

6. Abdellatiff H M, Burt B A. An epidemiological investigation into the relative importance of age and oral hygiene status as determinants of periodontitis. *J Dent Res* 1987; **66:** 13-18.

7. Bishop K, Briggs P, Kelleher M. Margin design for porcelain fused to metal restorations which extend onto the root. *Br Dent J* 1996; **180:** 177-184.

8. Lehner C R, Manchen R, Scharer P. Variable reduced metal support for collarless metal ceramic crowns: a new model for strength evaluation. *Int J Prosthodont* 1995; **8:** 337-345.

9. Sproull R C. Color matching in dentistry. Part II: Practical applications of the organization of color. *J Prosthet Dent* 1973; **29:** 556-566.

10. Moser J B, Wozniak W T, Naleway C A. Colour vision in dentistry: a survey. *J Am Dent Assoc* 1985; **110:** 509-510.

11. Culpepper W D. A Comparative study of shade-matching procedures. *J Prosthet Dent* 1970; **24:** 166-173.

12. Sorensen J A, Torres T J. Improved color matching of metal-ceramic restorations. Part I: A systematic method for shade determination. *J Prosthet Dent* 1987; **58:** 133-139.

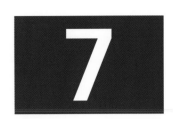

IN BRIEF

- Core placement nowadays demands more use of adhesives (coupled with retentive cavity preparation) and less use of pins
- It is good practice to remove existing restorations of unknown provenance to facilitate cavity inspection and ensure core retention
- Cores act either as a simple space filler or a structural build-up. The less tooth structure the greater the mechanical demands on the core, the material for which must be chosen carefully
- Dentists placing pins need to be aware of how to prevent and manage pin placement problems

Crowns and other extra-coronal restorations: Cores for teeth with vital pulps

R. W. Wassell[1] E. R. Smart[2] and G. St. George[3]

Cores for teeth with vital pulps is the seventh in the series of crowns and other extra-coronal restorations. A core is defined as 'that part of a preparation for an indirect restoration consisting of restorative material'. This article questions the need for routine pin placement and addresses the following issues — removal of existing restorations, the need for a core, core materials, core retention, and problem solving.

[1]*Senior Lecturer, [2]Lecturer, Department of Restorative Dentistry, The Dental School, Newcastle upon Tyne NE2 4BW [3]Specialist Registrar in Restorative Dentistry, Eastman Dental Hospital, 256 Grays Inn Road, London WC1X 8LD
*Correspondence to: Dr R.W. Wassell, Dept. of Restorative Dentistry, The Dental School, Newcastle upon Tyne NE2 4BW
E-mail: r.w.wassell@ncl.ac.uk

For almost half a century pinned amalgam restorations have been taught as the basis for cores in posterior vital teeth. Many schools, including our own, continue this venerable tradition in the knowledge that when skilfully carried out in optimal circumstances it seems to work well. However, clinical research on pin placement shows that the technique is not without problems.[1] Of 429 pin placements by staff and students at Leeds Dental School 19% showed complications — most frequently a loose pin or inadequate penetration of the pin into the pin channel. However, 10% of complications were serious involving either perforation of the pulp or periodontium, or tooth fracture. Inexperienced operators are especially prone to problems with almost half of the pins (41%) placed by second year students proving unsatisfactory. Experienced operators are not immune to difficulty; a survey of 37 practitioners placing 1394 pins over a 3-month period reported difficulties in 1 in 20 placements.[2]

A considerable amount of *in-vitro* evidence (see Table 1) shows the potential pins have for causing crazing of the dentine (look at Fig. 1) and pulpal sensitivity.

In addition, an animal study[12] showed severe pulpal inflammation where pins were placed within 0.5 mm of the pulp. Some self-shearing pins cause stressing and crazing when they 'bottom out' in the pin channel,[4] which may explain the symptoms some patients develop following pin placement. Of course, symptoms may also arise from undetected pulpal or periodontal perforations.

Fortunately there are other methods of retaining a core including the use of existing cavity preparation features, additional slots and boxes and, most importantly, adhesion. Much of the skill in placing a core involves the selection of the most appropriate material and technique, but whatever type of core is placed an important principle is that existing restorations should first be removed.

REMOVAL OF EXISTING RESTORATIONS

Figure 2 shows a tooth that clearly is a potential candidate for a crown. Only one cusp remains plus the remnants of another. The tooth has been repaired on a number of occasions and there is veritable jigsaw of amalgam 'fillings'. There is also a suggestion of mesial caries. No dentists in their right mind would pick up a handpiece and start to prepare this tooth for a crown. The most likely outcome would be a complete collapse of what is there with the potential for a rather difficult reassembly. Furthermore, if what is on display is representative of previous treatment, the possibility exists of there being residual as well as recurrent caries and even perhaps latent involvement of the pulp chamber.

Figure 3 shows a bitewing radiograph of the tooth. This adds to the diagnostic complexity of the case. What is holding the amalgam in place? There is no evidence of pins or other retentive devices and there are signs that the pulp chamber has been visited in the past. The clear evidence of dentine bridges indicate a successful pulpotomy and the question arises whether this should be accepted or in view of the potential risk of future pulp problems, should the tooth be root filled? (In this case the fillings were replaced with a more acceptable amalgam restoration and the tooth put on probation with a view to

Table 1. In vitro studies demonstrating problems with retentive pin placement

Problem	Reason for problem	Study
Crazing of dentine	Dulling of twist drill during pin channel preparation caused by an adherence of smear debris behind the drill's cutting edge.	Newitter et al., 1989[3]
	Stresses within dentine resulting from differences in diameter between the drill and the pin. Potential for damage increases with the number of pins inserted and . the pin diameter	Standlee et al., 1971[4] Kera et al., 1978[5]
	Pin placement strain caused by pins which have a core diameter (ie at the inner aspect of the thread) greater than the drill diameter	Bione and Wilson, 1986[6]
	Any fluid in the pin channel during pin insertion can contribute to cracking.	Hummert and Kaiser, 1992[7]
Pulpal inflammation following pin placement	Extensive cracks occurring with larger sized pins frequently communicate with the pulp chamber.	Webb et al., 1989[8]
	Heat generated during pin channel preparation, which is greater with larger diameter drills at higher speeds and deeper penetration.	Cooley and Barkmeier, 1980[9]
	Microleakage, which is worst with cemented pins and least with threaded pins. Cavity varnish does not reduce the problem	Chan, 1974[10]
	Some pins only partially penetrate the pin channel. This will reduce retention and leave a dead space prone to bacterial invasion.	Barkmeier and Cooley, 1979[11]

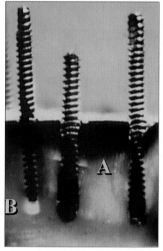

Fig. 1 Section of threaded pins placed into dentine. Notice the dentine crazing (A) and the failure of a pin to fully penetrate the pin channel (B)

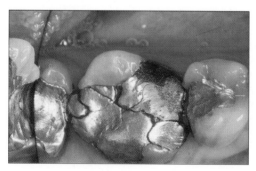

Fig. 2 Would you use this amalgam as a core?

re-assessing the endodontic condition and crowning it later.)

Before a crown preparation is undertaken, look closely at the tooth and form a mental picture of what will be left after cutting. Consider the existing restorations; decide on whether they are sound and whether they will remain in place during the cutting procedure. A history of the restoration should be determined but if this is not possible, especially if another operator has done the previous treatment, then consideration should be given to replacing the restoration. From personal experience, such restorations have been found on removal to have caries, cracked cusps and in some cases, latent pulp exposure beneath them. It is better to remove such fillings rather than be faced with an embarrassing endodontic emergency after the crown has been fabricated and cemented. It also gives you the chance to inspect (preferably under magnification) what remains of the tooth and decide whether this can be satisfactorily adapted to retain the core.

In summary, removal of existing restorations allows proper assessment of:

- The tooth's structural integrity (bearing in mind the need for mechanical core retention following tooth reduction during crown preparation)

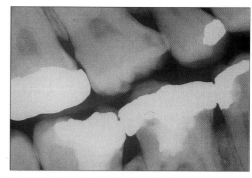

Fig. 3 Bitewing radiograph of tooth in Fig. 2 revealing a number of underlying problems

- Pulpal exposure
- Underlying caries

THE NEED FOR A CORE

It is useful to think of a core as either a 'build-up', which contributes significantly to the strength and retentiveness of the crown preparation, or 'filler' that simply alters the shape of the preparation, usually with the purpose of eliminating undercuts.[13] Fillers are often used on anterior teeth where class III and V restorations need to be replaced during tooth preparation.

Occasionally it may be necessary to electively devitalise a tooth and provide a post and core, often in combination with crown lengthening, to give adequate retention for the restoration (eg where only a root face exists). However a resin bonded indirect restoration may provide a viable alternative to devitalisation, especially where the intended crown is short occluso-gingivally. In this situation the adhesive would be subjected to less heavy peel and sheer stresses during function than if the crown were long.

It is worth emphasising that crown preparations do not always have to be built up with a core to an 'ideal shape'. Instead, existing cavity features can be refined to give suitable grooves and boxes. This approach is particularly useful for crown preparations affected by short clinical crown height (Fig. 4).

Cores may be placed either at the time of tooth preparation or beforehand. Where a patient requires only a single restoration the core and preparation can be made simultaneously in which case it is easiest to contour the core to resemble the intended preparation (Fig. 5). However, placing the core in advance gives a better opportunity to assess the integrity of a tooth and its pulp chamber and choose the most . appropriate indirect restoration for the amount and configuration of remaining tooth tissue. Cores placed in advance should be properly contoured to provide occlusal stability, patient comfort and freedom from food packing (Fig. 6). This approach becomes more crucial where patients require multiple cores. Once such cores are placed, the patient can be reviewed to ensure compliance with oral hygiene instruction, dietary advice and disease control. If the patient's response is unsatisfactory the provision

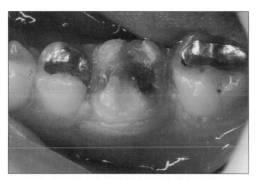

Fig. 4a A core is not always necessary. With teeth of short clinical crown height consider using internal preparation features rather than building up to a 'classical', textbook preparation

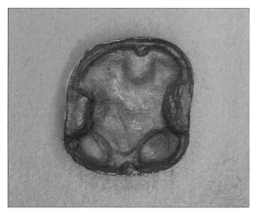

Fig. 4b The boxes and grooves of the preparation will be engaged by the fit surface of the crown providing a substantial increase in retention

of crowns may be suitably deferred. Core build-up materials need therefore to be chosen with care, as there is always the possibility that the core may in itself become the definitive restoration.

CORE MATERIALS
The material requirements of a core will differ depending on whether it is to be used as a build-up or filler. As a rule of thumb if sufficient tooth remains to provide a strong and retentive preparation then the core acts simply as filler. Should you be in any doubt it is better to choose a strong build-up material than risk mechanical failure of weak filler.

Amalgam
Advantages
- Not especially technique sensitive
- Strong in bulk section
- Sealed by corrosion products
- Can be 'glued' into place with cements and resins

Disadvantages
- Best left to set for 24 hours before tooth preparation
- Weak in thin section
- Mercury content may be of concern to some patients and dentists
- Potential electrolytic action between core and metal crown
- Not intrinsically adhesive

Recommendations
- Excellent core build-up material for posterior teeth
- Excellent interim restoration for posterior teeth
- Adhesives and preparation features can often substitute for pin retention

Amalgam has traditionally been regarded as the best build-up material under conventionally cemented crowns as it has good bulk strength and is sealed by its own corrosion products. It is not especially technique sensitive providing that during placement it is well condensed and is not grossly contaminated by blood or saliva. Although it is possible to find rapidly setting amalgams it is usually better to delay crown preparation for at least 24 hours.

Amalgam's main disadvantage lies in its mercury content which a minority of patients and dental practitioners find unacceptable. Also, the potential electrolytic action between the metal substructure of the future crown and the underlying amalgam is to some individuals a cause of concern[14] as it may liberate metallic ions. However, the intervening cement will act as an insulator and limit ion liberation, so unless the patient is suffering from lichen planus this is unlikely to be a problem.

Amalgam is weak in thin section and for this reason has no role to play in the provision of cores in anterior teeth. In posterior teeth the core may flake away if left in insufficient bulk following tooth preparation. Its retention is mainly mechanical, but increasingly adhesives are being used as will be discussed in the next section.

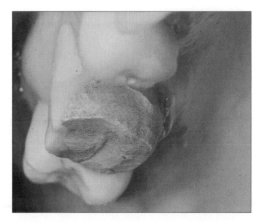

Fig. 5 It is sometimes convenient to build a core to resemble the intended preparation. (Courtesy of Professor Ian Barnes)

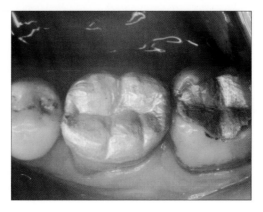

Fig. 6 Fully contoured cores are essential when longer-term interim restorations are needed

Composite

Advantages
- Strong
- Can be used in a thinner section than amalgam
- Fast setting (either light or chemically cured)
- Does not always need a matrix during placement
- Avoids mercury controversy

Disadvantages
- Highly technique sensitive
- Relies on multi-stage dentine bonding requiring effective isolation
- Dentine bond can be ruptured by polymerisation contraction
- Minor dimensional changes caused by the coefficient of thermal expansion (three times higher than the tooth) and water absorption — not usually clinically significant
- Can be difficult to distinguish between tooth and core during preparation

Recommendations
- Excellent build-up material for posterior and anterior teeth if isolation assured
- Aesthetic interim restoration, but takes far longer to place than amalgam
- Pin retention rarely necessary

Although composite is as strong as amalgam[15] it has only recently been accepted as a good core material, albeit a less forgiving one. Without dentine bonding agents microleakage[16] is a significant problem. Dentists who placed composite cores before the advent of dentine bonding agents will remember the resulting caries and pulpal problems — although surprisingly, this problem was never documented scientifically.

Effective bonds between composite and tooth are now possible, but only where moisture contamination and shrinkage can be properly controlled. The term 'wet bonding', whereby the dentine is left damp following etching and rinsing to encourage better penetration of the primer, should not lull us into a false sense of security. Experience shows blood and saliva contamination will render bonding useless. We therefore recommend the use of rubber dam and incremental placement of light cured composite to reduce shrinkage problems. Chemically cured composite can be placed as a single increment as shrinkage stresses are partially dissipated through the much longer setting time. Where

totally effective isolation cannot be achieved, as in many subgingival situations, the use of composite cores is contraindicated.

With an amalgam core there is usually little problem in identifying whether the finish line for a crown preparation lies on a core or on sound tooth tissue. With tooth coloured cores such discrimination can be difficult, even if a contrasting shade of composite is chosen. To overcome this difficulty composites have been introduced with titanium filler particles. These are chemically setting materials, which despite their impressively strong appearance have lower values of diametral strength, compressive strength and fracture toughness than regular light cured composite.[15,17] They are however stronger than GIC.

Glass ionomer

Advantages
- Intrinsically adhesive
- Fluoride release — but this does not guarantee freedom from 2° decay (Fig. 7)
- Similar coefficient of thermal expansion to tooth

Disadvantages
- Considerably weaker than amalgam and composite
- Tendency to crack worsened by early instrumentation
- Silver containing materials offer little improvement in physical properties
- Some materials radiolucent

Recommendations
- Excellent filler but relies on having sufficient dentine to support crown
- Where used as a build-up, best to leave tooth preparation until next appointment
- Good material on which to bond restorations with resin cement

Some dentists favour glass ionomers cements for cores, in view of the apparent ease of placement, adhesion, fluoride release, and matched coefficient of thermal expansion. Silver containing GICs[18] (eg the cermet, Ketac Silver, Espe GMbH, Germany) or the 'miracle mix' of GIC and unreacted amalgam alloy have been especially popular. Some believe the silver within the material enhances its physical and mechanical properties, however, *in-vitro* studies are equivocal[19,20] and a study of a cermet used to fill deciduous teeth showed that it performed less well than a conventional GIC.[21] In the days when many GICs were radiolucent, the addition of silver conferred radiopacity without which it would be difficult or impossible to diagnose secondary caries. Nowadays, many conventional GICs are radiopaque and are easier to handle than the silver containing materials. Nevertheless, many workers regard GICs as inadequately strong to support major core build-ups.[15,17,22–24] Hence the recommendation that a tooth should have at least two structurally intact walls if a GIC core is to be considered.[25] In our view it is best to regard GIC as an excellent filler but a relatively weak

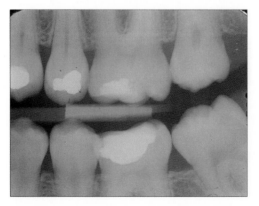

Fig. 7 GICs release fluoride, but this is not always effective in preventing decay as seen in this radiograph of a 10-year-old Ketac Silver core in the lower first molar

build-up material (Fig. 8). In order to protect a GIC core the crown margin should, wherever possible, completely embrace 1–2 mm of sound tooth structure cervically. Extension of the crown margin in this way is termed the 'ferrule effect'[26] and should ideally be used for all cores.

Resin modified glass ionomers

Advantages
- Command set
- Stronger than regular GICs
- Either intrinsically adhesive or with simplified bonding system
- Fluoride release

Disadvantages
- Most are weaker than amalgam and composite
- Hydrophilic resins cause swelling and can crack overlying porcelain
- Some materials can inhibit surface setting of addition silicone impressions
- Not reliable like amalgam and composite as an interim restoration

Recommendations
- Useful filler but confers few advantages over regular GIC

These materials come in a number of presentations, which can be used for a variety of purposes including fillings, cementation and core placement. They have been developed to provide properties intermediate between regular GICs and light cured composites. There is a spectrum of such materials. At one end are those that start to set in the same way as a GIC following mixing but are rapidly hardened by light curing the incorporated resin (eg Fuji II LC, GC International Corp, Leuven, Belgium). At the other end of the spectrum are the 'compomers', which have an initial setting reaction similar to composites (eg Dyract, Dentsply, Weybridge, UK). The GIC reaction does not occur until later when moisture from the mouth is absorbed into the set resin matrix where it activates incorporated polyacids. The resins used in these materials are hydrophilic and swell slightly following water absorption. This expansion has the potential to fracture ceramic restorations overlying cores and cements made with resin modified glass ionomers or compomers.[27]

Dentists have received these materials with some enthusiasm not least because the adhesive systems are easier to use than for composite resin and unlike GICs their rapid set does not delay tooth preparation. As well as good handling properties there is also the advantage of fluoride release.

Vitremer (3M, St Paul, USA) is an RMGI with good strength properties,[28] specifically advocated as a core material. In a short-term clinical trial it behaved satisfactorily under gold crowns, without the need for pin placement.[29] However, during the 3 months before crown preparation a third of the cores developed significant surface defects, which, although eliminated by crown preparation, suggest the material unsuitable for long-term interim restorations needed to estab-

lish occlusal stability. The authors were also at pains to emphasise the need for ferruling the crown preparation onto sound dentine in the same way as for regular GICs. Also of some concern, Vitremer prepared with a diamond bur had an inhibitory effect on the setting of a polyvinyl siloxane impression material.[30] This unset material may result in die inaccuracies.

At the present time we are not wildly enthusiastic about using these materials for cores other than as fillers.

CORE RETENTION

In this section we consider techniques of securing the core, which may be used either singly or in combination. These include:

- Cavity modifications
- Resin bonding
- Cement bonding
- Pins

There is little specific evidence of how well these methods work to retain cores but much information can be derived from laboratory studies and clinical studies of large amalgam or composite restorations.

Cavity modifications

Anyone who has had a core detach within a crown (Fig. 9) will know that it is unwise to place complete faith in either glues or pins. To gain mechanical retention for the core it is always worth capitalising on existing cavity features such as boxes or an isthmus. Where there is only a small amount of tooth tissue remaining it is also worth considering crown lengthening to ensure the crown margin is ferruled onto sound tooth structure.

Improved interlock between core and tooth can often be obtained by cutting new boxes or grooves, or by reducing and onlaying weakened cusps with core material. Where cusps are onlayed in this way the material must be sufficiently thick so that the core is not catastrophically weakened during occlusal reduction of the crown preparation. As a rough guide cusps should be reduced in height where they are less than 1 mm thick or the wall thickness to height ratio is less than 1:1.[31] Another useful tip is to resolve sloping walls into vertical and horizontal components. This approach will improve the resistance for both cores and castings. When cutting these auxiliary features one clearly wants to conserve tooth structure, but it is worth sacrificing non-critical amounts to make the work reliable. Problems with pulpal involvement may occur if such features are cut into the 'heart' of the tooth – a term used by Shillingburg[31] to describe the central volume of dentine beneath which lies the pulp. The heart may be avoided by not cutting any features more than 1.5 mm from the amelo-dentinal junction (ADJ) in a transverse plane.

Most dentists are familiar with the use of proximal grooves to retain Class II amalgam restorations. Not so many dentists know that

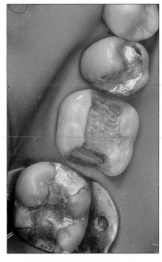

Fig. 8 GICs work best where the retention and resistance for the definitive restoration is derived mainly from surrounding tooth tissue. Here a silver cermet acts as excellent space filler in a gold onlay preparation

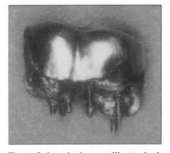

Fig. 9. A detached core still attached to its crown, despite a goodly number of pins. Notice that the crown does not provide a 'ferrule effect' and the absence of cavity retention features.

grooves can be used as an alternative to pins to retain large amalgam and composite restorations. Such grooves are cut into the base of cusps or into the gingival floor of boxes (Fig. 10). A small round bur (eg fi or 1 depending on tooth size) can be used. The depth of the groove needs to be sufficient to offer resistance to withdrawal of the head of the bur when it is used to gauge the presence of undercut. This usually means cutting to between two thirds and the complete depth of a round-headed bur. Grooves need to be positioned to within 0.5 mm of the amelo dentinal junction. Newsome has written an excellent account of the practical procedure.[32]

The use of grooves (sometimes termed 'slots') has been tested *in–vitro* and *in–vivo*. A circumferential groove used to retain a full coronal amalgam compared with four dentine pins showed no significant difference in dislodging force in one in-vitro study[33] but was less resistant in another.[34] The majority of pinned cores in these studies failed through amalgam slippage and pins bending. Where the slippage of amalgam had been slight this would have been difficult to detect clinically. By contrast failure of the grooved cores was all or none.

Short-term clinical trials show that groove retained amalgams perform at least as well as pinned amalgams.[35,36] However, grooves are associated with less pulpal inflammation than pins.[12]

The above studies were carried out *without* adhesives or dentine bonding. A combination of grooves and bonding should be even better.

Resin bonding
Resin adhesives were devised to bond composite restorations to enamel and dentine. These materials have been developed into luting agents for adhesively retained bridges and also bonding agents for amalgam restorations. Examples of amalgam bonding agents include:

Amalgam bonding agent	Adhesive resin
Panavia EX and Panavia 21	Phosphate ester of Bis GMA
All Bond 2	NPG GMA
Amalgam Bond and Amalgam Bond Plus	4 META/TBB-MMA, HEMA

In–vitro studies show that when properly placed these materials can enhance bond

strength[34,37–39] and reduce microleakage.[40] All Bond 2 has some of the highest bond strengths.[38] However, some bonding agents are ineffective, or relatively so, under conditions of *in–vitro* testing. For instance, Panavia 21 had such low bond strengths with one variety of amalgam it was considered ineffective for retention.[41] Worse still, all specimens made with Amalgam Bond debonded prior to testing.[38] But it needs to be emphasised that better results have been obtained with Amalgam Bond Plus[39,42] – a bonding agent, which provides a similar sheer strength to pin retained amalgams.[39,42] However mechanical retention, in the form of gooves or boxes,[43] should be provided where possible rather than rely entirely on the adhesive.[42]

A clinical study has also compared the performance of pinned amalgam restorations with those retained by resin adhesive. After 2 years both types of restorations performed equally well with no deterioration or loss of retention in either group.[44]

The disadvantage of most resin adhesives is that they require a multi-stage placement technique involving etching, washing, and priming before the amalgam is condensed onto the wet adhesive. Although some single-bottle primer/adhesive systems show promise for bonding amalgam,[45] extra time and effort is still needed and contamination during critical stages will destroy the bond.

Cement bonding (Baldwin technique)
Another way of getting amalgam to bond to dentine is to pack it onto a thin, wet layer of cement. This method, called the Baldwin Technique,[46] was reported in 1897 – the very same year as grooves were described.[47] Whilst this approach may seem old fashioned it should be remembered that screw pins for dentine also originated from that time.[48]

Baldwin used wet zinc phosphate cement to improve the seal of newly placed amalgam restorations. The technique never really caught on, possibly because traditional teaching insists that a cement base must be set to prevent its displacement by the condensed amalgam. Also, if zinc phosphate were extruded to the cavity margins in any thickness it would be vulnerable to dissolution. Nevertheless, wet cement has been recommended to assist with core retention by some highly reputable dentists.[49]

The evidence for using GICs as an amalgam core adhesive is currently only laboratory based. GICs form a good bond to dentine and an even better one to amalgam.[50,51] In bonding amalgam to dentine GICs and resins give similar results. Evaluations[37,52,53] have included shear, tensile and fracture strength tests for a variety of GICs (the luting agent, Ketac Cem; the base/lining material, Vitremer, and the filling material Fuji II).

Unfortunately there are no comparative data, either laboratory or clinical, to guide us in the selection of the most suitable GIC. Therefore, whilst the technique holds great promise we have to rely on empirical and derived informa-

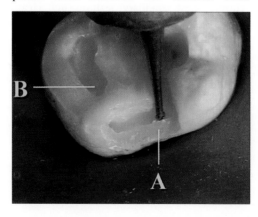

Fig. 10 Groove preparation in an upper molar. A fi round bur is being used to groove the cervical floor of the box. A: A number 1 round bur has been used in the lingual cusp B: Grooves should be sufficiently deep to offer some resistance to bur withdrawal

tion. For instance it would be best to avoid GICs designed for use as base materials, some of which have been shown to be soluble when used in the sandwich technique.[54]

Table 2 offers a clinical guide to using GIC as a bonding agent for amalgam.

Pins

It is not the purpose of this article to put pin manufacturers out of business, merely to draw attention to potential problems of pin placement and to emphasise viable alternatives. However, many dentists will still feel the need to place pins, perhaps on a belt and braces basis. Where the urge cannot be resisted the advice in Table 3 may help reduce problems.

PROBLEM SOLVING

Many, although not all core placement problems relate to the use of pins. Problems with pins can be avoided by using alternative techniques.

Inadequate isolation

Cores are often required for heavily broken down teeth with subgingival involvement where oozing gingival margins cause problems with visibility, caries removal and moisture control. At the simplest level a well-placed matrix band along with cotton wool rolls and aspiration may provide sufficient isolation, but not always. Rubber dam too may fall short of providing excellent isolation. However, spaces between tooth and rubber can be remedied by syringing in a caulking material such as Ora Seal Putty (Optident Ltd, Skipton, UK). This material must be kept clear from the cavity margin. Electro-surgery can be used first to remove any gingival excess and gingival bleeding controlled with a styptic agent such as Astringident (Optident Ltd, Skipton, UK).

Pin in periodontium or pulp

One event guaranteed to leave most dentists hot under the collar is when the drill suddenly gives and the patient gives a cry of pain or blood oozes out of the pin channel. Alternatively the pin continues to worm its way in, perhaps perforating a thin dentine wall separating the pin channel from either pulp or periodontium. Such perforations can be difficult to treat and before taking action it is important to first confirm the site of the perforation. A periapical radiograph may help, but an electronic apex locator, which will read 'beyond the apex' if the pin or pin channel is in the periodontium, will give an instant and reliable diagnosis.[57] For both periodontal and pulpal perforations the important principle of treatment is to prevent microbial ingress. Treatment decisions are necessarily empirical in the absence of controlled clinical studies.

Periodontal perforations are perhaps most difficult to remedy and if left can result in chronic infection and long-term patient discomfort. A perforation within the gingival sulcus should be included within the margin of

Table 2 The Baldwin Technique modified for use with GIC cement and amalgam
• Optimise mechanical retention with grooves, boxes etc.
• Use Vitremer or a GIC luting agent with a longer working time
• To prevent the set cement from sticking to the matrix band apply a thin layer of petroleum jelly to its inner aspect. This must be done before fitting the matrix band or the cavity will be contaminated
• Ensure good isolation but do not over-dry the cavity as this may result in post operative sensitivity
• Apply a thin layer of cement over the entire cavity surface
• Condense the amalgam into the deepest areas first (eg boxes and grooves) encouraging the wet cement to be extruded up to the occlusal surface
• When the cavity has been packed full remove the last increment of cement-contaminated amalgam and repack with a fresh increment

Table 3 How to reduce pin placement problems

Pin selection

• Avoid large pins for initial pin placement as they are not significantly more retentive than medium pins

• Select a pin with a stop to prevent 'bottoming out', and a buttress thread to maximise retention (Fig. 11) and minimise dentine stress[55] (eg Unity Pins, Whaledent, Mahwah, USA)

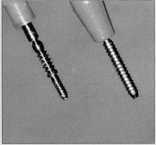

Number and location of pins

• Restrict the number of pins – normally no more than one per missing cusp

• Place pins in locations non-hazardous to pulp and periodontium:

  • 1 mm from the ADJ

  • Towards the corners of molars[56]

  • Avoiding the central palatal area in upper molars (risk of pulp perforation of the palatal root)

  • Avoiding the centre of proximal boxes, especially in maxillary first premolars and other teeth with proximal root concavities (Fig. 12)

  • Avoiding areas apical to the cemento-enamel junction

Fig. 11 The pin on the left has many desirable features. In particular, notice the stop half way along its length to prevent it 'bottoming out' in the pin channel. The rounded contours above the stop are designed to reduce stress concentration in the core

Pin channel preparation

• Ensure the twist drill is not dull and runs in the correct direction

• Angulate the pin drill by aligning it against the outer surface of the tooth

• Run drill at moderate speed without excessive pressure

• Partially withdraw drill after cutting the first 1 mm to allow debris to clear

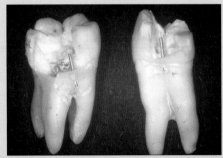

Fig. 12 Pins can easily perforate the periodontium in areas of root concavity of molars and premolars

Pin placement

• Use a speed reducing hand piece or run the hand piece at low speed

• Use low pressure and let the pin find its way in

• If necessary, bend the pin inwards to ensure clearance between the pin and matrix band

the intended restoration or else it will become a subgingival plaque trap. A crown lengthening procedure involving gingivectomy or raising a flap (if necessary with bone recontouring) is usually needed to access the pin. The pin can then be either trimmed level with the root surface[1,58] or the open perforation sealed. If the pin has been placed into the periodontal ligament it may be possible to remove it ultrasonically from the coronal aspect, although with a freshly placed pin this can take considerable time.[59] If the pin can be removed the new root canal perforation sealant, MTA (Mineral Trioxide

Aggregate, Dentsply, Tulsa, USA), has the potential to provide an excellent, biocompatible seal.[60] The occlusal portion of the pin channel may need to be opened up sufficiently to allow moisture control and the material to be condensed properly. If the pin is not retrievable it may be left and the tooth put under probation with a view to later crown lengthening surgery should the tooth give symptoms. Certainly, it would be unwise to place an expensive indirect restoration on such a tooth until its prognosis was confirmed.

Pulpal perforations are usually easier to manage than periodontal perforations. Many teeth requiring large cores have a questionable pulpal status, and, if perforated are best root treated, especially if the tooth is crucial to the treatment plan and the outcome of the root treatment can be assured. However, if there is no rush to provide an indirect restoration the tooth can be kept under probation and a pulp capping technique used. Many materials seem well tolerated by the pulp providing a bacteriological seal can be established and maintained. Some authorities suggest that even the pin itself can act as a 'pulp cap'[61,62] but few dentists sterilise their pins before placement and the space between dentine and the inner diameter of the thread will allow bacteria to spiral down into the pulp. At the very least the pin and surrounding dentine will need to be surface sealed with a dentine-bonding agent. Alternatively, the pin may be removed ultra sonically (if it has already been placed) and the pulp capped with calcium hydroxide or MTA,[60] followed by sealing with composite and dentine bonding agent.

Of course, groove preparation also has the potential to perforate either the pulp or periodontium, but this is likely to be a less frequent event than pin perforation and should it occur access for repair is very much easier.

Loose pin
A pin may become loose immediately after placement, during pin length reduction or whilst replacing an old pin retained restoration. If a medium sized pin has been used it can be replaced with a large pin. Alternatively, the wisdom of replacing the pin can be reviewed, the pin channel converted into a groove and the core bonded adhesively.

A pin that is too tall will protrude through the occlusal surface of the core. Where the pin is shortened with a bur it can very easily come unscrewed, especially if the bur is kept in line with the pin, which causes an anticlockwise frictional force. The chatter from a tungsten carbide bur is also effective in dislodging pins. We recommend holding the tip of a long tapered diamond bur at right angles to the pin and cutting from the side rather than grinding from above. An airotor handpiece should be used with a light touch. In this way the frictional forces generated tend to act on the pin in a clockwise direction. Needless to say this procedure should be done with water coolant and with aspiration to catch the fragment of cut pin.

Tooth fracture during pin placement
Root treated or brittle teeth can chip and fracture especially if the pin is placed too close to the ADJ. It emphasises that dentine is deformed by pin placement resulting in stresses which can crack the tooth. If the tooth can be saved, the fractured area should be covered by the restoration.

Matrix band placement
The placement of a matrix band can often prove a challenge to even the most experienced of dentists. However, ensuring the proximal contacts are open and that there are no spicules of tooth at the gingival margin can facilitate placement. The choice of band is highly personal and the best matrix system is 'the one which works best for you.' However occasions arise when a more sophisticated matrix system is needed, such as the Automatrix system (LD Caulk Co, Milford, USA), which has the advantage of not being encumbered by a matrix retainer. In common with other systems it does need to be wedged and where there are multiple cusps to be replaced it may sometimes need to be stabilised using greenstick, taking precautions not to scald the patient with hot composition.

Despite great advances in operative dentistry the copper ring (PD Copper Bands, Vevey, Switzerland) is sometimes the only way of fitting a matrix to a tooth, especially where all the cusps have been lost. It is best to choose a band that is, if anything, slightly too small, trim it to size with Bee Bee scissors and squeeze it to the approximate outline of the tooth. It can then be adapted section by section around the tooth stretching the band slightly with an amalgam plugger or half Hollenback instrument. If the band is too tight to fit it can be annealed and stretched further. Annealing involves heating the copper to cherry red heat in a gas flame and quenching. Although many would consider leaving such a band in place to allow the amalgam to be supported whilst it sets there is a risk of unseen, excess material being left and this could lead to gingival inflammation. It is usually an easy matter to slit the band with a tapered diamond bur and remove it at the time of placement. Orthodontic bands or aluminium temporary crown shells with their occlusal surfaces removed can act as a substitute for copper rings,[63] but aluminium reacts with mercury to form a flocculent airborne precipitate.

Early core fracture
We have all had the frustration of early core fracture occurring whilst the matrix band is removed or when the patient bites onto a partially set amalgam. If only a small portion of the core breaks away it is often possible to shape the remaining amalgam to provide a retentive cavity and pack fresh amalgam – sometimes without the need for the matrix being replaced. A more

PFM the amount of tooth preparation may be reduced slightly by using a special metal composite coping (Captek, Schottlander, Letchworth, UK). This type of coping is 0.1–0.2 mm thinner than a cast coping made from a noble metal alloy.

Composite crowns which use newly developed laboratory materials have not been fully evaluated. Specific indications and limitations have yet to be defined. Manufacturers are currently recommending that the tooth be prepared in the same way as for a HSPC.

The major factor to be considered before selecting the most suitable type of crown is the amount of tooth destruction you are willing to allow in order to give the aesthetics you want. You may also want to consider the need for the crown to incorporate special features, for example:

- A metal anterior guidance surface
- Rest seats and other features to retain a partial denture
- Metal occlusal surfaces for a bruxist

GUIDELINES FOR AMOUNT OF TOOTH REDUCTION AND MARGIN DESIGN

Tooth preparation represents a balance between, conserving tooth structure and pulp health on the one hand, whilst on the other, achieving an aesthetic and strong crown. Guidelines for the amount of tooth reduction for different types of crown have evolved largely as a result of experience rather than scientific evidence. Tables 2 and 3 give an indication of the amount of occlusal and cervical reduction for different types of crowns for posterior and anterior teeth. It is worth emphasising that there will be times when less tooth should be removed in the interests of conserving tooth structure and pulp health. There are also occasions when little or no tooth reduction is needed, eg from the occlusal surface when the vertical dimension is to be increased, or, from the buccal surface where the tooth is already worn and is to be re-contoured by the crown.

The amount of reduction can be gauged using depth cuts coupled with a knowledge of the appropriate bur end diameter (look at Fig. 4 for examples of typical bur end diameters). A preparation reduction matrix, formed on a diagnostic wax-up (described in the sixth article in the series), can be invaluable when the shape of the intended crown differs from that of the original tooth.

The metal margins of VMCs and PFMs can be configured in a variety of ways (Fig. 5). It is best to avoid the knife edge as the finish line can be difficult for the technician to detect. Chamfer margins and shoulder with bevel margins allow a fine edge of metal to be cast which, if a suitable alloy is chosen, can be burnished by the technician to improve marginal fit. However, there is always the danger that the die may be damaged by burnishing. Furthermore, the margin should

Table 2 Suggested preparation features for posterior crowns

Crown type	Posterior crowns — preparation features	
	Occlusal reduction*	Finish line depth and configuration
VMC	1 mm non-functional cusps	0–1.0 mm
	1.5 mm functional cusp	Chamfer, knife-edge,
		shoulder or shoulder with bevel
HSPC	2 mm non-functional cusps	0.8–1.0 mm
	2.5 mm functional cusps	Shoulder or heavy chamfer
PFM	As for VMC if metal surface	1.2 mm labial shoulder[†] or chamfer
	2 mm non-functional cusps	0.5 mm lingual chamfer
	2.5 mm functional cusps	

*Where tooth is tilted or where vertical dimension is to be increased, the amount of occlusal reduction required will vary

[†]Too deep a reduction for diminutive teeth or for long clinical crowns where a metal collar is preferable

Table 3 Suggested preparation features for anterior crowns

Crown type	Anterior crowns — preparation features	
	Occlusal reduction*	Finish line depth and configuration
PJC	2 mm incisally	0.8–1.0 mm shoulder
	1 mm lingual aspect	
RBPC	2 mm incisally	> 0.4 mm chamfer
	0.5–1.0 mm lingual aspect	
PFM	2 mm incisally	1.2 mm labial shoulder[†]
	0.5–1.0 mm lingual aspect	or heavy chamfer
	(porcelain guidance requires greater clearance)	0.5 mm lingual chamfer

*Where the vertical dimension is to be increased, the amount of occlusal reduction required will be less or non-existent

[†]Too deep a reduction for diminutive teeth eg lower incisors or for long clinical crowns where a metal collar is preferable

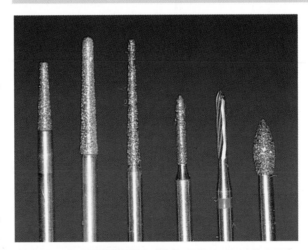

Fig. 4. Burs used for preparation of full veneer crowns at Newcastle Dental Hospital (from left to right): a) Flat-end tapered diamond (occlusal and axial reduction) end Ø = 0.8 mm; b) Long, round-end tapered diamond (as for a. and also shoulder production) end Ø = 1.1 mm; c) Long needle diamond (initial proximal reduction); d) Chamfer diamond (chamfer production) end Ø = 1.0 mm; e) Chamfer tungsten carbide (chamfer and preparation finishing); and f) Large flame or 'rugby ball' diamond (lingual concavity production)

not be too acute. Theoretical arguments have been made in favour of acute margins compensating for seating discrepancy[4] but only before cementation. Once cemented, an acutely bevelled margin may prevent the crown from seating fully,[5,6] presumably by restricting cement extrusion.

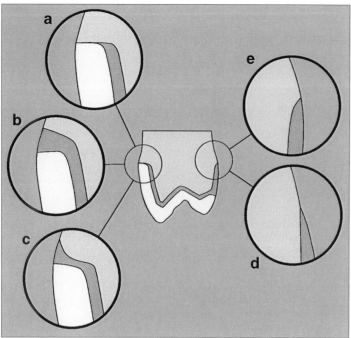

Fig. 5. Finish lines with marginal configurations for PFMs: a) Shoulder with porcelain butt fit; b) Deep chamfer with metal collar; c) Shoulder plus chamfer (bevel) with metal collar; d) Knife edge with metal margin; and e) Chamfer with metal margin

ceramic and metal margins. This approach can produce acceptable results for metal margins, although it is easier for the technician to adapt the wax and finish to a chamfer. A much greater problem occurs when ceramics are used as the inevitable consequence is for the crown to be over-bulked resulting in compromised aesthetics and a poor gingival emergence profile.

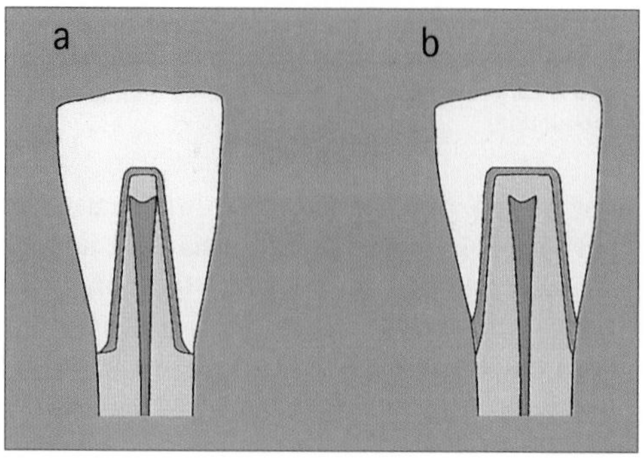

PREPARATION TAPER

The subject of taper is contentious. In the first place it means different things to different people. For our purpose it has the same meaning as 'convergence angle' ie the angle between opposing preparation walls. To avoid confusion when reading different publications, it is important to appreciate that 'taper' may also be defined as 'the angle between a single preparation wall and the long axis of the preparation'. Taper defined by the first definition will be twice the angle defined in the second.

As regards the question of ideal convergence angle, text books have traditionally based their recommendations (variously between 3 and 14°)[7-9] on the results of experimental studies[10,11] which show a decrease in retention of conventionally cemented crowns as taper is increased. Experimental studies have also shown that preparations with tapers greater than 20° display a significant fall in resistance to oblique displacing forces[12] and show increased stress concentration within the cement[13] which may rupture the cement lute.

On the other hand, clinical measurements of taper have been made indirectly on stone casts.[14-18] These studies showed mean values of about 20° with a considerable variability around the mean. Furthermore, greater tapers were achieved on mandibular molars than on maxillary incisors[19] possibly because of differences in tooth shape and problems with access. These findings suggest that clinicians, even those who are technically gifted, frequently cut a greater taper than text books recommend.

The issue of taper may not be quite as critical for single crowns as was once thought, but as a working rule operators should strive to produce the least taper compatible with the elimination of undercut. It is helpful to know that many tapered burs have a 5–6° convergence angle which can be used to survey preparation taper by holding the handpiece in the same plane for all axial surfaces.

Resin bonded crowns are the important exception to the rule of minimizing taper, especially RBPCs which may benefit from having tapers of about 20° to avoid generating high seating hydrostatic pressures during luting resulting in crown fracture.

As a general rule when using porcelain or PFMs, adequate clearance is required to achieve good aesthetics. Traditionally, this is achieved with a shoulder or heavy chamfer of 0.8–1 mm width for PJCs and 1.2 mm width for PFMs. However, shoulders of these depths may compromise tooth strength and pulp health especially for diminutive teeth such as mandibular incisors. A similar problem occurs on teeth with long clinical crowns because of the narrowing of their diameter in the cervical region. In a long preparation extending onto or beyond the cemento-enamel junction, considerable tooth tissue must be removed to eliminate undercuts. Solutions include using a minimal shoulder, a metal collar on a chamfer (as illustrated in Fig. 6) or placing the margin at the cemento-enamel junction. Under normal circumstances these options do not compromise aesthetics, being hidden by the lip. Clearly, patients need to understand the benefits of a less destructive preparation and, as stated previously, must be involved in the decision making process pre-operatively.

Some operators use what they describe as a mini-shoulder, 0.5–0.7 mm wide, for both

STRATEGIES FOR ENHANCING RESISTANCE AND RETENTION

While many factors influence resistance and retention, one of the most important is the nature of the cement lute. Conventional cements are strong in compression and weak in

Fig. 6. Teeth with long preparations are prone to pulpal exposure especially if a deep finish line is cut. (a) Teeth with narrow roots are most vulnerable (b) A metal collar reduces the need for a deep finish line

tension, so, wherever possible, preparations should be designed to limit tensile and shear stresses in the lute, especially when oblique forces are applied to the crown (Fig. 7). Cement selection will be considered in detail in Part 11 of the series.

Preparations which are either short or over-tapered or both are vulnerable to crown dece-mentation. Often one is confronted with having to replace a crown where the preparation is over tapered and simply re-preparing the tooth may be excessively destructive. This section considers aspects of preparation design and other methods which can be used to prevent decementation.

Any dentist who has seen a number of dece-mented crowns will have an idea of what an unretentive preparation looks like. However, there are no absolute guidelines for preparation dimensions which risk decementation. An *in-vitro* study[20] has shown a significant increase in resistance and retention as axial walls extend from 2–3 mm in height and recommended 3 mm as the minimum preparation height. As a working rule this seems reasonable but there will be a multitude of exceptions and caveats depending on factors such as taper, cement selection and occlusal loading.

Where the preparation is over-tapered it is possible to up-right the axial walls at the base of the preparation, but this can result in a deep shoulder, excessive destruction of tooth tissue and possible compromise of pulpal health. If the bulk of remaining core or tooth tissue permits, a series of near parallel steps can be made in the over-tapered axial walls which results in a much less destructive preparation.

Other less destructive approaches of dealing with an unretentive preparation are:

- Retentive preparation features ie grooves and boxes
- Resin cements
- Surgical crown lengthening
- Pins and cross-pinning

Grooves and boxes provide increased reten-tion by presenting additional near-parallel sided walls to the preparation and limiting the path of insertion. Resistance is improved by preventing rotation of the restoration (Fig. 8). They are used mainly for metal and metal-ceramic restorations but are generally impractical for all ceramic crowns.

Grooves

Grooves can be placed in one or more of the axial walls using a minimally tapered bur. The bur chosen should be of sufficient diameter to provide a groove that will not be blocked out on the die with die-spacer (see flat-end tapered dia-mond in Fig. 4). The groove should be placed within a sound bulk of tooth tissue or core not leaving any weak surrounding areas which are liable to fracture. The tooth may also be less vul-nerable to the effects of micro-leakage if the base of the groove is kept 0.5 mm clear of the

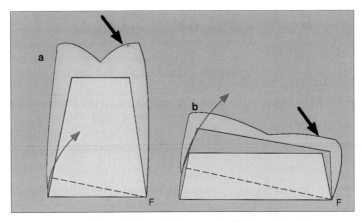

Fig. 7 Preparations (a) and (b) have similar retention (similar axial surface area and convergence angle) but (a) has much greater resistance. Application of oblique force to occlusal surface results in potential rotation of crown (a) around a fulcrum (f). Rotation is resisted by the cement above the arc of rotation of the base of the crown being thrown into compression — represented by arrow. Rotation of the shorter crown (b) results in tensile forces fracturing the cement lute. It is therefore important that the radius of rotation intersects the opposing axial wall.[28]

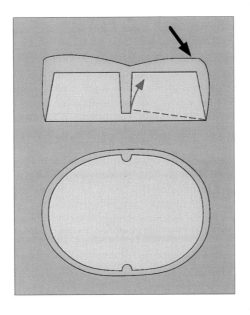

Fig. 8 Placement of axial grooves increases resistance by effectively reducing the radius of rotation

finish line. To be effective the groove should be sunk to at least half the bur's diameter. When placing grooves in tapered axial walls be very careful to ensure that the walls of the groove do not conflict with the path of insertion. This requires the bur to be held parallel to the path of insertion and not parallel with the tapered axial wall. Providing these precautions are taken, grooves provide a simple, effective means of improving resistance.

Boxes

Boxes function similarly to grooves in providing increased resistance and retention, but are less con-servative so it is difficult to justify them being cut into sound tooth structure unless there are other reasons for their presence (eg provision of a crown with an intra-coronal attachment). Nevertheless, a tooth may have previously contained a restoration with a box form. Instead of using the box to retain a core the box can be incorporated into a crown preparation. This is a useful approach where the core would otherwise be thin and weak. You may need to take care to ensure the resulting crown is not so bulky that casting porosity or thermal sensitivity becomes a problem.

Boxes need not necessarily be sited solely on axial walls For example, it is sometimes very useful to cut an intra-coronal box, resembling an occlusal inlay, into the occlusal aspect of a substantial core. Clearly, this approach would be inappropriate if it weakened the core appreciably.

Resin cements

Resin cements (to be described in Part 13 of the series) provide a relatively simple option to overcome the low tensile strength and poor adhesion of conventional cements. Resin cements have much higher tensile strength[21] and when used in combination with dentine bonding agents are less sensitive to repetitive dislodging forces.[22,23] They are, however, technique sensitive and are not supported by long term clinical data. Current clinical wisdom is, where possible, to combine sound retentive design with resin cementation.

Crown lengthening

Exposure of a greater height of clinical crown may involve either gingivectomy (with a scalpel or electrosurgery) or flap surgery with osseous recontouring. It is an invaluable means of enhancing retention, but can be a substantial undertaking and has to be balanced against the disadvantage of patient discomfort. Details of technique are described elsewhere.[24] Crown lengthening needs to be planned in advance of tooth preparation (Fig. 9). If the ultimate position of the gingival margin is critical then good provisional restorations should be provided and worn for 2–3 months before the final impression

to allow the gingival tissues to recover fully to their final form.

Pins and cross-pins

Pins and cross pins are rarely used as they are technically demanding and have become even less popular since the introduction of resin cements. Pins may be considered where there is a good bulk of tooth tissue. They are incorporated during the construction of the restoration and are sunk through the occlusal surface.

Cross-pins are placed following cementation and are screwed transversely through the axial surface of the crown into the underlying preparation.

TOOTH PREPARATION

To avoid any unwanted surprises, the structural, endodontic, periodontal, aesthetic and occlusal factors outlined in the previous parts of the series should be checked before bur is put to tooth.

There are a variety of burs which can be used for crown preparations and operators will have their own preferences. Some operators may prefer a flat ended bur for shoulder production. However, the round ended bur has the benefit of producing a rounded junction between the finish line and axial walls which will help reduce stress concentration in this vulnerable part of the preparation and is less likely to cut steps.

Most practitioners in the UK use air rotor handpieces, although in continental Europe and elsewhere speed increasing handpieces are favoured. Whatever option is chosen a water spray is absolutely essential to avoid

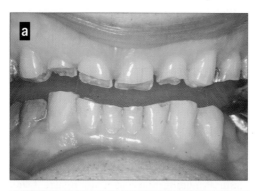
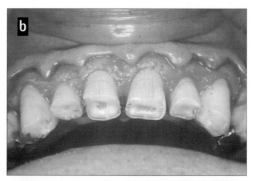
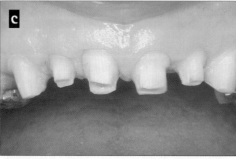
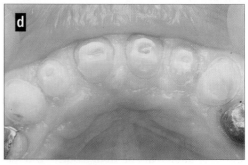

Fig. 9 When clinical crown height is short, plan ahead. a) Upper anterior teeth needing crowning with PFMs b) Crown lengthening using apically repositioned flap and osseous recontouring c) Preparations made 3 months after surgery. Note no incisal reduction needed as vertical dimension to be increased d) Preparations viewed occlusally (mirror view) showing retention grooves in cingulum of UL2 (22)

pulpal damage and endodontic complications. Following air rotor preparation, a speed increasing handpiece can be useful for finishing the preparation, defining finish lines and placing retention devices such as grooves or boxes.

Preparation sequence

There are definite advantages in following a set order of tooth reduction and ensuring that each element of reduction is complete before starting the next. For instance, if the occlusal surface is prepared first there will be better access for the more difficult proximal preparation. Depth cuts placed before embarking on larger areas of tooth reduction help ensure controlled removal of tooth tissue but where the proposed crown is to be shaped differently from the original tooth a preparation matrix, as described in Part 6 of the series, is more helpful. During axial preparation it is best to complete the most difficult wall first so if any alignment modifications are required they can be made in more accessible areas.

Each stage of reduction has its own special considerations and these will now be discussed in the sequence of preparation that we would recommend.

Posterior preparations

Occlusal reduction

Before any reduction is carried out it is important to assess the occlusion and note any space already available between opposing teeth. For example, a mesially tilted molar may require little or no reduction of its mesial occlusal surface so depth cuts can be confined to the distal occlusal area. If the reduction follows the cuspal contours you will get maximum axial wall height available for resistance and retention, but clearly this is not so critical where long axial walls are to be prepared. The functional cusp bevel, shown in Fig. 10, is a useful feature of the occlusal reduction and ensures space for adequate bulk of crown material in a site of heavy occlusal contact. The functional cusp (or holding cusp) must be identified and, after bevelling, adequate clearance should be confirmed in all excursive movements. This small simple step helps avoid the creation of an occlusal interference or perforation of a crown's occlusal surface.

Lingual reduction

Lingual access may be difficult. However if the lingual surface is the first axial surface to be prepared, it reduces the likelihood of producing an over tapered preparation especially if the bur is held parallel to the long axis of the tooth. Subsequent alignments to the prepared lingual wall are then carried out on more accessible surfaces.

Buccal reduction

Good retention relies on near parallelism cervically of the buccal and lingual axial walls. However, it is also important to ensure that the preparation is in harmony with the buccal contours of the adjacent teeth so that sufficient

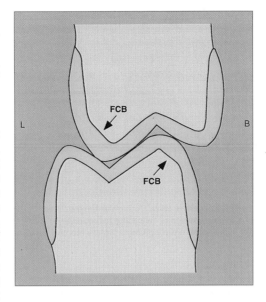

Fig. 10 Functional cusp bevel (FCB) of the holding cusps required for occlusal clearance

space is available for good aesthetics. It is worth viewing the tooth from both occlusal and buccal aspects to ensure the correct planes of adjustment have been made.

On molars the preparation may extend towards the furcation region where a concavity of the buccal surface can be found. To avoid creating a crown with an over-bulky buccal surface, the finish line should be cut to its full depth in this area and the concavity should be extended up the buccal axial wall to the occlusal surface. This approach, which may also need to be used on other axial walls with cervical concavities, eg the mesial aspect of upper first premolars, results in a preparation having a kidney shaped appearance when viewed occlusally.

Proximal reduction

During proximal reduction many adjacent teeth are damaged.[25] If a fine tapered bur is used for the preliminary cut it can be kept safe by ensuring a fine sliver of tooth or core material remains between the preparation and the adjacent tooth. This sliver can then be flicked away before refining the reduction with a bur of larger diameter. To ensure clearance of the proximal contact, try to keep the tip of the bur at the level of the proposed finish line. There is no doubt that this is the most difficult stage of the preparation.

Once the basic preparation is complete, check the path of insertion and taper. Again, if you view the preparation from both occlusal and buccal aspects you should ensure that no undercut goes undetected. A surface reflecting mirror is especially useful for such inspection. When viewing occlusally do so with one eye closed because an undercut can be perceived as a near parallel taper when seen with two eyes. Take special care to check the junction between proximal and buccal/lingual reductions which are a common site for undercuts.

On PFM preparations, where the deeper reduction for porcelain and metal meets the shallower reduction for metal (this is shown from the occlusal aspect in Fig. 3a) there is often a distinct step in the axial wall. This feature is termed

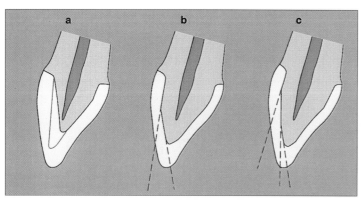

Fig. 11 Single plane reduction (a) can result in either shine through of the porcelain core (feint outline) or pulpal damage. Problem solved by two plane reduction (b). Three plane reduction (c) needed for long clinical crowns giving a slightly more buccal path of insertion

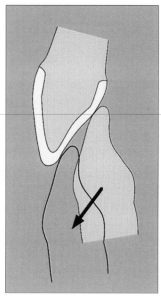

Fig. 12 Ensure occlusal clearance in both ICP and excursions

rather confusingly the 'wing', resulting in generations of students creating a bizarre preparation resembling a small bird in flight, but correctly cut it is a useful feature providing some increase in resistance and helps guide the technician in the position of the porcelain-metal junction. Should a metal proximal contact be required the 'wing' should lie buccal to the contact. Conversely, if a porcelain proximal contact is planned the wing should lie lingual to the contact. To avoid undercut it is important that the wing is made parallel to the buccal axial reduction.

Finish line

Ideally, this should be placed supra-gingivally[26,27] on sound tooth tissue, but in reality this is often not possible. Sometimes aesthetics dictates a margin is placed subgingivally and in these situations it should extend by 0.5–1 mm, but certainly no more than half the depth of the gingival sulcus, to ensure the epithelial attachment is not compromised. Packing of retraction cord in the gingival sulcus prior to preparing the finish line will allow displacement of the gingival margin for access and help minimise gingival trauma during preparation. Whether a finish line should ever be placed on core rather than tooth is an area of contention. Some consider the practice acceptable if the core has a perfect margin. However, in practice it is rarely possible to guarantee the condition of the core margin and we would generally recommend the preparation should be extended sub-gingivally to finish onto sound tooth tissue. Where the finish line is likely to be extensively sub-gingival a crown lengthening procedure can often facilitate crown provision and ensure a more accessible crown margin.

Whatever type and location of finish line is chosen it is important that:

• It has no unsupported lips of tooth structure at the edge which can either break away on the die causing problems with crown seating or break away from the tooth resulting in a marginal gap. Use hand instruments to plane these away
• It is in harmony with the outline of the gingival margin which will optimise aesthetics of crowns finished at or above gingival level, and, for sub-gingival margins, will ensure there is no localised over-cutting
• The technician will be able to detect it on the die
• There is sufficient space to provide a crown with an appropriate gingival emergence profile.

Additional retention features

At this stage consider whether, as described earlier, there is a need for grooves or boxes to enhance resistance and retention in a short or tapered preparation.

Final finishing

Complete smoothing of the preparation is not essential, may diminish micro-mechanical retention and may also risk overheating the pulp if it is not done under water spray. However, the final preparation must be free from irregularities, sharp line angles and corners. These cause difficulty in casting models and result in dies which are vulnerable to damage leading to an ill-fitting crown. An area which is often neglected is the axio-occlusal line angle but it is important that all line angles and corners are carefully rounded. This is especially so for preparations for all ceramic restorations to reduce areas of potential stress concentration.

Anterior preparations

With the exception of provision of a functional cusp bevel, anterior preparations need similar consideration to posterior preparations. However, a few additional points need highlighting:

• Incisal reduction is best carried out first. This will improve subsequent preparation access and helps to ensure correct proportioning of axial reduction planes
• The reduction of the labial surface should be in two or more planes to achieve good aesthetics and conserve tooth tissue. Long clini-

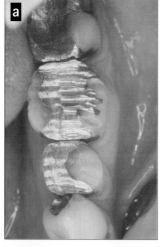
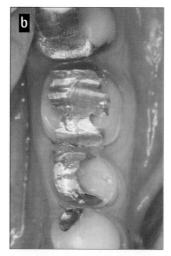

Fig. 13 Full veneer crown preparation LL6 (36) and three quarter preparation at LL5 (35): a) Occlusal reduction carried out on both teeth. In the same way each axial surface was completed sequentially. Note the depth grooves on the occluso-buccal aspect of LL6 (36); b) The completed preparations showing the mesial finish line on a sound amalgam core

cal crowns will often need to undergo three plane reduction; Figure 11 illustrates this

- The palatal reduction needs to reproduce the natural concavity of maxillary teeth if space is to be provided for the development of anterior guidance; Figure 12 illustrates this. Unless clearance during lateral and protrusive movements has been checked, it is very easy to end up with a crown which occludes satisfactorily in the intercuspal position, but which interferes during excursions.

Multiple preparations

Preparation of multiple teeth can be stressful for both patient and dentist. Where possible try to sequence treatment so that no more than four teeth are prepared at one sitting or perhaps six if dealing with the maxillary anteriors.

If you are able to prepare multiple teeth with a mutual path of insertion it will facilitate the construction of provisional restorations and helps with cementation of definitive crowns. However, this must not be done at the expense of excessive tooth reduction. To ensure a mutual path of insertion it is usually best to prepare each surface sequentially for all the teeth rather than fully complete each preparation before moving onto the next (Fig. 13).

CONCLUSION

Crown preparations are destructive to underlying tooth tissue and can affect the pulp. Therefore, the type of crown selected should have the least destructive preparation in keeping with the patient's functional and aesthetic requirements. Where appropriate the use of less destructive, adhesively retained restorations should be considered.

The authors would like to thank Mr Alan Waller, Audio-Visual Department, for help with the diagrams. Thanks also to Drs Eoin Smart and Ian Macgregor for their constructive criticism and careful proof reading.

1. Shillingberg H T, Hobo S, Whitsett L, Jacobi R, Brackett S E. *Fundamentals of fixed prosthodontics.* 3rd ed. Chicago: Quintessenence, 1997.
2. Burke F J T. Fracture resistance of teeth restored with dentin-bonded crowns: the effect of increased tooth preparation. *Quintessence Int* 1996; **27:** 115-121.
3. Broderson S P. Complete-crown and partial-coverage tooth preparation designs for bonded cast ceramic restorations. *Quintessence Int* 1994; **25:** 535-539.
4. Rosner D. Function placement and reproduction of bevels for gold castings. *J Prosthet Dent* 1963; **13:** 1160-1166.
5. Ostlund L E. Cavity design and mathematics: Their effect on gaps at the margins of cast restorations. *Operative Dent* 1985; **10:** 122-137.
6. Gavilis J R, Morency J K, Riley E D, Sozio R B. The effect of various finish line preparations on the marginal seal and occlusal seat of full crown preparations. *J Prosthet Dent* 1981; **45:** 138-145.
7. Dykema R W, Goodacre C J, Phillips R W. Johnston's Modern *Practice in Crown and Bridge Prosthodontics.* pp.24. Philadelphia: W.B. Saunders Co., 1986.
8. Shillingburg H T, Hobo S, Fisher D W. *Preparations for Cast Gold Restorations.* pp.p16. Chicago: Quintessence Publishing Co., 1974.
9. Tylman S D, Malone W F P. *Tylman's Theory and Practice of Fixed Prosthodontics.* pp.103. St. Louis: C. V. Mosby Co., 1978.
10. Jorgensen K D. Relationship between retention and convergence angle in cemented veneer restorations. *Acta Odontol Scand* 1955; **13:** 35-40.
11. Kaufman E G, Coehlo D H, Colin L. Factors influencing the rentention of cemented gold castings. *J Prosthet Dent* 1961; **11:** 487-502.
12. Dodge W W, Weed R M, Baez R J, Buchanan R N. The effect of convergence angle on retention and resistance form. *Quintessence* 1985; **16:** 191-194.
13. El-Ebrashi M K, Craig R G, Peyton F A. Experimental stress analysis of dental restorations. Part III. The concept of the geometry of proximal margins. *J Prosthet Dent* 1969; **22:** 333-345.
14. Ohm E, Silness J. The convergence angle in teeth prepared for artificial crowns. *J Oral Rehabil* 1978; **5:** 371.
15. Eames W B, O'Neal S J, Monteiro J, Roan J D, Cohen K S. Techniques to improve the seating of castings. *J Am Dent Assoc* 1978; **96:** 432.
16. Mack P J. A theoretical and clinical investigation into the taper achieved on crown and inlay preparations. *J Oral Rehabil* 1980; **7:** 255.
17. Norlander J, Weir D, Stoffer W, Ochi S. The taper of clinical preparations for fixed prosthodontics. *J Prosthet Dent* 1988; **60:** 148-151.
18. Noonan J E, Goldfogel M H. Convergence of the axial walls of full veneer crown preparations in a dental school environment. *J Prosthet Dent* 1991; **66:** 706-708.
19. Kent W A, Shillingburg H T, Duncanson M G. Taper of clinical preparations for cast restorations. *Quintessence Int* 1988; **19:** 339-345.
20. Maxwell A W, Blank L W, Pelleu G B. Effect of crown preparation height on the retention and resistance of gold castings. *Gen Dent* 1990; May-June: 200-202.
21. Michelini F S, Belser U C, Scherrer S S. Tensile bond strength of gold and porcelain inlays to extracted teeth using three cements. *Int J Prosthodont* 1995; **8:** 324-331.
22. Wiskott H W, Nicholls J I, Belser U C. The relationship between abutment taper and resistance of cemented crowns to dynamic loading. *Int J Prosthodont* 1996; **9:** 117-139.
23. Wiskott H W, Nicholls J I, Belser U C. The effect of tooth preparation height and diameter on the resistance of complete crowns to fatigue loading. *Int J Prosthodont* 1997; **10:** 207-215.
24. Smith D G. Toothwear: Crown lengthening procedures. In: Barnes I E, Walls A W G, editors. *Gerodontol* pp.109-117. Oxford: Wright, 1994.
25. Moopnar M, Faulkner K D. Accidental damage to teeth adjacent to crown-prepared abutment teeth. *Aust Dent J* 1991; **36:** 136-140.
26. Silness J. Periodontal conditions in patients treated with dental bridges. II. The influence of full and partial crowns on plaque accumulation, development of gingivitis and pocket formation. *J Perio Res* 1970; **5:** 219-224.
27. Silness J. Periodontal conditions in patients treated with dental bridges. III. The relationship between the location of the crown margin and the periodontal condition. *J Perio Res* 1970; **5:** 225-229.
28. Hegdahl T, Silness J. Preparation areas resisting displacement of artificial crowns. *J Oral Rehabil* 1977; **4:** 201-207.

Details of burs mentioned in article		
Bur	No	Supplier
Flat-end tapered diamond	554	Kent - AD Burs Ltd, Gloucester, UK
Long, round-end tapered diamond	503	Kent - AD Burs Ltd, Gloucester, UK
Long needle diamond	557	Kent - AD Burs Ltd, Gloucester, UK
Chamfer diamond	877/010	Komet-Brasseler gmbh, Lemgo, Germany
Chamfer tungsten carbide	282/101	Komet-Brasseler gmbh, Lemgo, Germany
Large flame ('rugby ball') diamond	257/023	Horico-Hopf Ringled & Co GmbH, Berlin, Germany

- The functions of provisional (sometimes termed temporary) restorations
- Diagnostic uses of provisional restorations
- Provisional restorations for conventional preparations including: the concept of short, medium, and long-term temporisation; materials; and direct and indirect provisional restorations
- Provisional restorations for adhesive preparations
- Problem solving

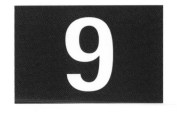

Crowns and other extra-coronal restorations: Provisional restorations

R. W. Wassell[1] G. St. George[2] R. P. Ingledew[3] and J. G. Steele[4]

The important role of provisional restorations is often overlooked. This may be because they are left until the end of an appointment when time for construction is short or because they generally do not need to last for long. However, not only can good provisional restorations help produce better final restorations, they can also save a lot of time and expense at subsequent appointments. In fact time spent in their construction will be more than repaid in time saved doing additional procedures, adjustments and remakes later on.

[1],[4]Senior Lecturer in Restorative Dentistry, Department of Restorative Dentistry, The Dental School, Newcastle upon Tyne NE2 4BW; [3]Senior Dentist, Boots Dental Care, 54-58 High Street, Maidenhead, Berkshire SL6 1PY; [2]Higher Specialist Trainee, Eastman Dental Hospital, 256 Grays Inn Road, London WC1X 8LD
*Correspondence to: Dr R. W. Wassell, Department of Restorative Dentistry, The Dental School, Newcastle upon Tyne NE2 4BW
E-mail: R.W.Wassell@newcastle.ac.uk

This article discusses the need for provisional restorations, the types and materials available. Provisional restorations for adhesive restorations often pose a difficult problem and these are considered separately. You may also encounter other difficulties with provisional restorations so we end the article on problem solving.

Functions of provisional restorations

Provisional restorations are used in the interim between tooth preparation and fitting a definitive restoration. The various functions they fulfil are described in Table 1. With crown preparations provisional restorations are generally essential to cover freshly cut dentine and prevent tooth movement. With adhesive preparations protection of exposed dentine is usually less of an issue and often a provisional restoration is not needed, but there are still occasions where it is important to prevent unwanted tooth movement or maintain aesthetics.

Provisional restorations can be invaluable for testing out aesthetic and occlusal changes before they are incorporated in the definitive restoration. They can also help stabilise the periodontal condition prior to definitive restoration. These diagnostic uses will be considered in more detail in the next section.

As well as the prophylactic and diagnostic uses, provisional restorations have other practical applications. For example, callipers may be used to test the thickness of a provisional restoration to ensure sufficient tooth preparation to accommodate the proposed restorative material (Fig. 1). Occasionally, a provisional restoration may be used to provide a coronal build up for isolation purposes during endodontic treat-

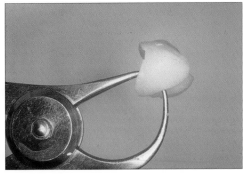

Fig. 1 Provisional restorations have many functions other than just protection of the prepared tooth. Here an Svensen gauge is used to assess sufficient tooth reduction to accommodate the proposed restoration

ment. A period of long-term provisional restoration may also be advisable to assess teeth of dubious prognosis. Finally, a provisional restoration may find a use as a matrix for core build ups in grossly broken down teeth, simply by removing the coronal surface to allow placement of restorative material.

DIAGNOSTIC USES

Provisional restorations, especially those used for conventional preparations, are invaluable in situations where aesthetic, occlusal or periodontal changes to a patient's dentition are planned. The principles behind such changes are discussed later.

Aesthetic changes

Proposed changes to the shape of anterior teeth are best tried out with provisional restorations to ensure patient acceptance, and, approval from friends and family; clearly, it is easier to trim or add acrylic than it is porcelain. Once happy, an

Table 1 The functions of provisional restorations

1) Comfort/tooth vitality	To cover exposed dentine to prevent sensitivity, plaque build up, subsequent caries and pulp pathology.
2) Occlusion and positional stability	To prevent unwanted tooth movement by the maintenance of intercuspal and proximal contacts. It may be necessary to establish a holding contact on the provisional restoration. Depending on the patient's occlusal scheme, the provisional restoration may need to provide guidance in protrusive and lateral excursions, or disclude to prevent working or non working interferences. Interproximal contacts also need to be maintained to prevent food packing.
3) Function	Attention to 1) and 2) will ensure the patient continues to function adequately.
4) Gingival health and contour	To facilitate oral hygiene and prevent gingival overgrowth provisional restorations require accurate margins and cleansable contours. They can be used in the interim where the level of the gingival margin has yet to stabilise (e.g. after crown lengthening or removal of a crown with defective margins).
5) Aesthetics	To provide an adequate interim appearance provisional restorations should either mimic the tooth just prepared, or the final intended restoration.
6) Diagnosis	To assess the effect of aesthetic and occlusal changes. The ability to re-shape can also be used to overcome phonetic problems before construction of the definitive restoration.
7) Other practical uses	To measure tooth reduction, to isolate during endodontics, to assess prognosis, to act as a matrix for core construction.

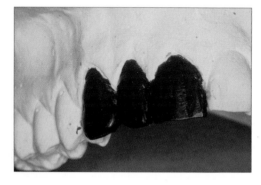

Fig. 2 A diagnostic wax-up is an invaluable way of planning changes, which can be tried out with the provisional restorations. The patient would be more impressed by tooth coloured wax!

alginate is recorded so that the technician can copy the shape into the definitive restoration. If only one or two teeth are involved it is perfectly possible to contour provisional restorations at the chair side. It is however important to balance the time spent doing this against the advantages of having a diagnostic wax up and matrix made in the laboratory (Fig. 2). Alternatively, indirect provisional restorations can be prescribed which will be described later.

Occlusal changes

A patient's tolerance to changes in anterior guidance or increased occlusal vertical dimension is best tried out with provisional restorations. Again, a diagnostic wax up is advisable, and, with occlusal changes, the importance of using casts mounted on a suitable articulator cannot be overstated (Fig. 3). Direct or indirect provisional restorations are then constructed from these and cemented temporarily after adjusting to provide even occlusal contact in the intercuspal position and guidance or disclusion if required. The patient can then be examined at a further appointment and the occlusal surfaces copied as long as the following criteria are met:

- Restorations are still cemented
- Occlusal contacts have been maintained, with no drifting of teeth
- Teeth are not mobile, or existing mobility is not increasing
- There is no discomfort

Guidance surfaces can be copied between provisional and definitive restorations by using a custom guidance table as described in Part 5 of the series.

Where it is decided to increase the patient's occlusal vertical dimension, provisional restorations provide a way of assessing tolerance to the increase, as well as assessing aesthetics and the overall occlusal scheme. However it is often wise to make an initial assessment of such changes with a more reversible method, such as a splint, before the teeth are prepared.

Periodontal changes

It may be necessary as part of a patient's periodontal treatment to remove overhanging restorations to allow access for cleaning and resolution of inflammation. Long-term wear of properly fitting and contoured provisional restorations allows the health of the gingival margin to improve and its position to stabilise before impressions are recorded for definitive restorations.

Following periodontal or apical surgery the tissues will also need time to stabilise before the final finish line is cut for definitive crowns. Where surgical crown lengthening is used to increase clinical crown height, it is best to allow 6 months before definitive restoration, especially if the aesthetics are critical.[1] If provisional restorations are provided soon after crown lengthening it is important to avoid taking the preparations subgingivally as this may set up a chronic gingivitis which is difficult to resolve.

Changes in tooth shape — avoiding problems

For the majority of people, minor adjustments in tooth shape are unlikely to cause any problems, but for others, eg singers and wind instrument musicians, the eventual restorations, if poorly planned, may interfere with the patient's 'embouchure'. This term describes the fine mouth movements and lip/tooth contact required for speech production or sound generation in the case of a musical instrument. Also the incorpo-

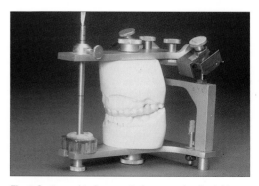

Fig. 3 Casts need to be mounted on a semi-adjustable articulator to wax occlusal changes

ration of wider cervical embrasure spaces, to facilitate interproximal cleaning, may occasionally cause embarrassment because of air leakage. Therefore it makes sense to copy the features of successful provisional restorations, to avoid patient dissatisfaction and expensive remakes.

PROVISIONAL RESTORATIONS FOR CONVENTIONAL PREPARATIONS

The variety of provisional restorations available can seem bewildering. To help you through the maze we need first to consider the materials and then the techniques by which provisionals can be made. Most provisionals are made directly at the chair side, but for long term wear or diagnostic use there can be advantages in having them laboratory-made.

It is worth emphasising that the length of time between preparation of teeth and cementation of final restorations can vary from a few days for straightforward cases (short-term), to several weeks (medium-term) or even, in the case of complex reconstruction, several months (long-term). The longer provisional restorations are in the mouth, the greater are the demands on the material from which they are made.

Materials

Materials used in the surgery comprise pre-formed crowns (made of plastic or metal), self cured or light cured resins or resin composites and cements. Laboratory formed temporaries are generally made in self cured or heat cured acrylic, or cast metal.

Pre-formed crowns

Also known as proprietary shells, these come in a series of sizes but usually need considerable adjustment marginally, proximally and occlusally. Plastic shells are made from polycarbonate or acrylic, and, with good aesthetics, are commonly used for anterior teeth including premolars. Metal shells may be made from aluminium, stainless steel or nickel chromium and are only used on posterior teeth. Both plastic and metal shells can be relined with self cured resin to improve their fit.

Self or light cured resins

A variety of materials is available for either direct or indirect techniques:

- Polymethyl methacrylate (self or heat cured) (eg Vita K&B Acrylics)
- Polyethyl methacrylate (eg Snap, Trim)
- Bis acryl composite (eg Protemp, Quicktemp)
- Urethane dimethacrylate (light cured) (eg Provipont DC)
- Restorative composite

Polymethyl methacrylate is strong, has a high wear resistance, is easy to add to, and has good aesthetics, which is maintained over longer periods.[2] However, it does have three main disadvantages:

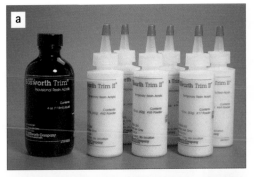

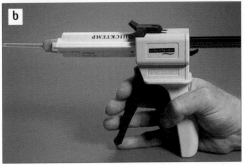

Fig. 4 Examples of resins used for provisional restorations: (a) Polyethyl methacrylate (powder-liquid presentation); and (b) Bis-acryl composite (syringe mixed)

i) Polymerisation shrinkage which can affect fit
ii) Polymerisation exotherm which can damage pulp[3]
iii) Free monomer may cause pulp and gingival damage

It is, however, a good material for indirect provisional restorations. Self cured acrylic can be polymerised under pressure in a hydroflask which effectively reduces porosity.[4] Alternatively, heat cured acrylic can be used.

Polyethyl methacrylate (Fig. 4a) is suitable for intra-oral use as it shrinks less and is less exothermic than polymethyl methacrylate. However, strength, wear resistance, aesthetics and colour stability are not as good. Some presentations come with a good colour range (eg Trim II) while others have only light and dark shades (eg Trim).

Bis-acryl composites (Fig. 4b) produce less heat and shrinkage during polymerisation than other resins, resulting in a better marginal fit.[5] Despite being reasonably strong they are brittle in thin section and difficult to add to. Aesthetically they are reasonable, but few shades are available and they stain easily if the unpolymerised surface layer is not removed which may be accomplished with alcohol and polishing. They are more colour stable than polyethyl methacrylate materials and are therefore better suited for use as long-term provisionals.[6]

Most recently, visible light cured resins have been introduced based on urethane dimethacrylate eg Provipont D.C. These relatively expensive resins have good mechanical properties and, being light cured, the operator has some control over the material's working time. Generally more shades are available than bis acryl composite and the colour is relatively stable, but is still prone to staining. Marginal fit can be poor,

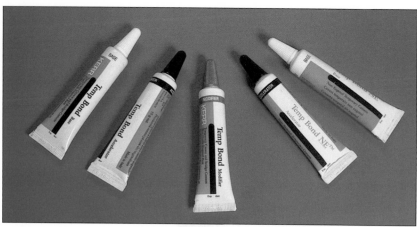

Fig. 5 Temp Bond and Temp Bond <u>NE</u>: The modifier (central tube) can be mixed with Temp Bond Base and Catalyst to ease crown removal with retentive preparations. Regular Temp Bond contains eugenol, which can soften composite cores. Temp Bond <u>NE</u> (shown to right of photograph) does not contain eugenol and will avoid this problem

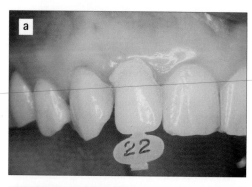

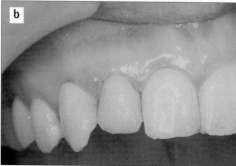

Fig. 6 (a) A familiar polycarbonate shell crown relined with Trim; and (b) The provisional is carefully trimmed to help maintain gingival health

Provisional cements

Provisional restorations are usually cemented with soft cement. Traditionally, a creamy mix of zinc oxide eugenol was used, but nowadays most dentists prefer proprietary materials such as Temp Bond (Fig. 5). This material comes with a modifier, which is used to soften the cement, as described later in the article, to ease removal of the provisional restoration from more retentive preparations. Temp Bond <u>NE</u> is a non-eugenol cement which may be used for patients with eugenol allergy or where there is concern over the possible plasticising effect of residual eugenol on resin cements and dentine bonding agents. Certainly, surface hardness[11] and shear bond strength of resin[12] to resin can both be affected by eugenol and it is worth noting that eugenol cements can significantly reduce the bond of resin cements to composite cores.[16] However, resin bond strengths to enamel[13] and dentine[14] are not affected if the eugenol residue is removed with pumice and water before conditioning. Microleakage[15] is also unaffected by the use of eugenol.

Occasionally, hard cement is needed to retain a provisional on a short preparation. This is considered later in the 'problem solving' section.

Direct provisional restorations — techniques

Most provisional restorations will be made directly in the mouth. As mentioned earlier it is worth taking time in their construction. As a rule of thumb, the time taken to temporise a tooth should be similar to the time taken to prepare it. This approach ensures sufficient time is devoted to good fit and contour. The techniques available are listed overleaf:

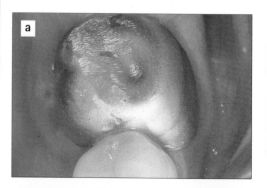

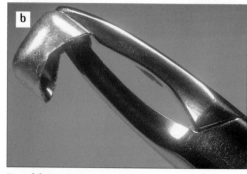

Fig 7 (a) Aluminium shell crowns are convenient, but suitable only for short term use on posterior teeth; and (b) Crimping of the crown margins will improve retention and fit

but the material can be added to. Light cured materials, especially unfilled ones, have a higher exotherm than chemically cured materials because of their greater speed of reaction.[7] This exotherm may have implications for pulpal health.

Restorative composites, normally used for filling teeth, can be used as a provisional material for adhesive preparations, as described later. Other restorative composites are designed for laboratory fabrication but may be useful for long-term provisional restorations.

Cast metal

Alloys used include nickel chromium, silver and scrap gold. Copings can be cast with external retention beads for acrylic or composite. In less aesthetically critical areas of the mouth, metal may be used on its own. Cast metals are very durable, but rarely used unless provisional restorations have to last a long time.

- Shells (proprietary or custom)
- Matrices (either formed directly in the mouth or indirectly on a cast)
- Direct syringing

To avoid confusion with terminology, a shell is incorporated into the provisional restoration whereas a matrix is merely used to form it.

Proprietary shells
Shells can be divided into proprietary and custom made. Proprietary shells made of plastic (Fig. 6) or metal (Fig. 7) are used commonly in practice when only one or perhaps two preparations are involved.

Proprietary plastic shells: A crown with the correct mesio-distal width is chosen and placed on the tooth preparation. The cervical margins are trimmed to give reasonable seating and adaptation. The preparation is then coated with petroleum jelly and the crown, containing a suitable resin eg Trim, is reseated. While the resin is still incompletely set, the proximal excess is removed using a sharp bladed instrument such as a half Hollenback amalgam carver. The crown is then removed and replaced several times to prevent resin setting in undercuts. Finally, the crown is adjusted and polished using steel or tungsten carbide burs and Soflex discs. Diamond burs are best avoided, as they tend to melt the shell and resin because of the heat generated.

Proprietary metal shells: Aluminium crowns are really only suitable for short-term use as they are soft resulting in wear and deformation. Furthermore, they can produce galvanic reactions in association with amalgam restorations. Their fit is usually poor unless considerable time is spent trimming and crimping the margins followed by relining with a resin. Stainless steel or nickel chromium crowns may occasionally be used on molar teeth opposed by flat cusps where heavy occlusal loading would quickly wear or break a resin crown.

Custom shells
Some operators favour custom shells for multiple tooth preparations. The shell is made in advance of tooth preparation so the desired external contours are pre-formed, but relining and careful marginal trimming are necessary prior to fitting. Custom shells are of two types, either beaded acrylic or 'Mill Crowns'. Both offer the advantage of being able to use the superior properties of polymethyl methacrylate, whilst avoiding pulpal damage by constructing the shell out of the mouth.

The beaded acrylic shell is formed within an impression taken of the teeth prior to preparation or of a diagnostic wax up. A thin shell of polymethyl methacrylate is constructed in the impression by alternately placing small amounts of methyl methacrylate monomer followed by polymer, taking care not to make the shell too thick, otherwise it will need time-consuming adjustment later. Once set, it is trimmed and then relined in the mouth as with polycarbonate crowns.

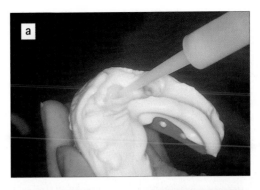

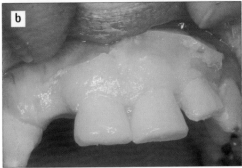

Fig. 8 (a) A commonly used matrix is an alginate impression of the unprepared tooth; and (b) The flash must be removed and the linked provisionals trimmed prior to cementation

Mill Crowns are formed by first cutting minimal crown preparations on a stone cast. A pre-preparation matrix is then filled with polymethyl methacrylate and placed over the preparations. The trimmed and adjusted provisional crowns are again relined in the mouth.

Matrices
Many operators prefer matrices (Fig. 8) to shell crowns for making single or multiple provisional crowns. This is because matrices closely duplicate the external form of satisfactory existing teeth, or, if changes are required, a diagnostic wax up. If the matrix is carefully seated minimal adjustments are generally needed other than trimming flash at the crown margin.

There are three main types of matrix:

- Impression (alginate or elastomer)
- Vacuum formed thermoplastic
- Proprietary celluloid

The simplest way of making a matrix is to record an impression of the tooth to be prepared either in alginate or silicone putty. Impression matrices are quick, easy and inexpensive, and can be formed while the local anaesthetic is allowed to take effect. When impression matrices are used some judicious internal trimming may be helpful to improve seating and bulk out critical areas of the provisional restoration. These aspects are covered later when we deal with problem solving. Alginate matrices are best at absorbing the resin exotherm[3] – although the temporary should have been removed before this stage of set. Elastomeric impression matrices have the advantage of being reusable, allowing them to be disinfected and stored in case they are required again. Polyvinylsiloxane putty impressions are frequently used because of their ease of handling and long-term stability.

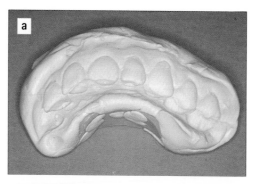

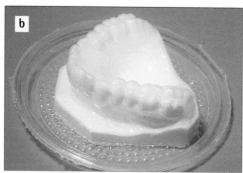

Fig. 9 Where aesthetic or occlusal changes are proposed, provisional crowns can be formed in the mouth with laboratory-made matrices: (a) A putty or alginate matrix can be formed directly on the wax–up (remember to soak cast first); and (b) A vacuum formed matrix can also be made, but on a stone duplicate of the wax-up to prevent the wax from melting (matrix shown prior to trimming)

If a tooth is broken down or its shape needs to be changed, it will first need to be built up. Soft red wax can be used for this purpose, but anyone who has tried this will know that it does not stick well. Adhesion can be improved dramatically by first painting the tooth with a coat of varnish (eg copal ether or glass ionomer varnish) and allowing it to dry. The opposing teeth are smeared with petroleum jelly to allow their form to be stamped into the wax should it be necessary to build up the occlusal surface. Rather than try and achieve perfection with an intra-oral wax-up it is better to aim for a slight over-contour, which can be corrected by trimming the provisional restoration. It is best to avoid putty for making the matrix as it can distort or displace the wax when the impression is seated.

There is no doubt that the above technique is invaluable, however, when dealing with multiple crowns it is a much better strategy to first carry out a diagnostic wax up on mounted casts (Fig. 3). The intended aesthetics and occlusion can be formed much more efficiently and patients appreciate being able to see a 'blue print' of the definitive restorations on the articulator. Moreover, the wax up can be used to form a suitable indirect matrix.

Indirect matrices can be made from impression material (Fig. 9a) or you can ask your laboratory for a vacuum formed matrix made of clear plastic (Fig. 9b). If you decide to make an indirect matrix from impression material remember to first soak the cast for five minutes. In this way you will avoid the embarrassment of sticking impression to cast. Immersion in warm water (not hot) has the advantage of speeding up the impression material's setting time.

Vacuum formed matrices are made of clear vinyl sheet produced on a stone duplicate of the waxed up cast. This is necessary to avoid melting the wax when the hot thermoplastic material is drawn down. Not everyone is enthusiastic about using a vacuum formed matrix because they are flexible and can distort when seated, especially if there are few or no adjacent teeth to aid location. Where it is necessary to rely on the soft tissues for matrix location we prefer to use an impression matrix.

Whilst vacuum formed matrices are not without problems, being made of clear plastic they are indispensable for moulding light cured resins. A proprietary celluloid matrix can be used if only a single provisional crown is to be formed using light cured resin.

Whatever matrix is chosen care must be taken in its use. After tooth preparation, a thin smear of petroleum jelly is placed over the reduced tooth and adjacent teeth. The matrix is blown dry and the mixed resin is syringed into the deepest part of the appropriate tooth recess, taking care not to trap air, especially at the incisal angles. After reseating, the matrix is left until the resin reaches a rubbery stage. It is then removed and interproximal excess removed in the same way as for the proprietary shell. Setting can be monitored to some extent by testing the consistency of a small portion of material syringed onto the front of the seated impression. Following removal, the crowns are trimmed, polished and cemented.

Direct syringing
When no shell temporary can be found to fit and, for whatever reason, no matrix is available it can be useful to syringe material directly around a preparation. For this purpose the poly-ethyl methacrylate materials are best as they can be mixed to sufficient viscosity not to slump but are still capable of being syringed. This property whereby a material undergoes an apparent decrease in viscosity at high rates of shear, as when passed through a syringe nozzle, is called 'shear thinning'. It is also seen with the polyether material, Impregum.

When syringing, start at the finish line and spiral the material up the axial walls. Overbuild the contours slightly as it is easier to trim away excess than to have to add later.

Indirect provisionals
Many dentists will not have used indirect provisional restorations and may find it hard to justify laboratory costs. However, indirect provisionals offer certain advantages with complex cases needing long-term temporisation. Firstly, materials which are stronger and more durable can be used eg heat cured acrylic or self cured acrylic cured in a hydroflask. Secondly, if aesthetic or occlusal changes are to be made these can be developed on an articulator. Indirect provisionals can certainly save clinical time, especially with multiple restorations and most particularly where there is to be an increase in vertical dimension, especially where the patient is a bruxist (Fig. 10).

Whether or not major changes are indicated, it is best to decide on the type of provisional restoration during treatment planning. If indirect restorations are chosen, sufficient time can be scheduled either to make them whilst the patient waits or an additional appointment can be made to fit those made in the laboratory.

Some operators favour making indirect provisional restorations from self cured acrylic at the same appointment the teeth are prepared. If the surgery has an on site technician (or suitably trained nurse) this can be a very efficient way of working as it allows the dentist to do something else while the provisional restorations are being made. An alginate impression is recorded of the prepared teeth and this is cast up in quick setting plaster. The plaster model is then coated with cold-mould seal and a suitable shade of self cured acrylic mixed up. The acrylic is then flowed into a matrix made from the diagnostic wax up (eg silicon putty or vacuum formed) which is then seated onto the cast and its position stabilised with elastic bands, taking care not to distort it. Polymerisation takes place within a hydro flask following which the matrix is removed; the relatively soft plaster dug out and the acrylic flash trimmed back to the margin. Additions may need to be made to the margins of the crowns where polymerisation shrinkage has produced a gap. This can be done in the mouth or on a cast. If done in the mouth, then the tooth needs lubricating with petroleum jelly and the crowns removed before excessive heat is generated.

Clearly, an extra appointment will be necessary if indirect provisional restorations are made in an outside laboratory. In the interim direct provisional restorations will also be needed. This approach can be very effective, however, where an increase in vertical dimension is prescribed. A number of strategic teeth can be prepared and interim provisional restorations made directly to conform to the existing occlusion (eg from polyethyl methacrylate or Bis acryl composite). On return, the indirect provisional restorations can be used to establish the increased vertical dimension on multiple teeth. Often these cases require minimal or no occlusal preparation as occlusal clearance is provided by the increase in vertical dimension. When this happens the interim provisional restoration will resemble a tube with no occlusal surface, which is usually acceptable for short periods.

PROVISIONAL RESTORATION OF ADHESIVE PREPARATIONS

Provisional restorations for conventional tooth preparations (eg full veneer crowns, 3/4 crowns, and onlays) obtain retention in a similar way to the final restorations ie via cement on preparations with long, minimally tapered axial walls. The lack of conventional retention provided by most adhesive preparations results in temporary cements being ineffective. A number of strategies can be used to deal with this problem, some

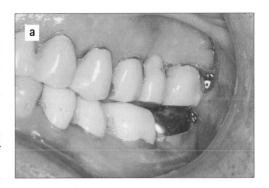

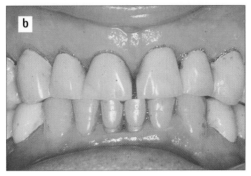

Fig. 10 Metal and acrylic provisionals used in the occlusal reconstruction of a bruxist: (a) A relined NiCr shell at tooth LL7 (37) where the previous acrylic provisional crown had fractured repeatedly; and (b) The upper arch has acrylic heat cured onto beaded metal copings in an attempt to improve fracture resistance — however a good bond between metal and acrylic is needed for success

of which are more appropriate for certain situations than others:

- No temporary coverage may be necessary eg with veneer preparations involving minimal dentine exposure and not removing intercuspal or proximal contacts. Where space has been created with a Dahl appliance, the appliance can be used in the interim to retain the teeth in position
- A simple coat of zinc phosphate cement to protect exposed dentine eg in tooth preparations which are not aesthetically critical and where the occlusion is either not involved or the restoration can be returned rapidly from the laboratory and fitted before significant tooth movement occurs
- Composite resin bonded to a spot etched on the preparation eg veneer preparations which are aesthetically critical or occlusally critical or have sensitive, fresh cut dentine. The provisional restoration is fabricated using either directly placed composite which is time consuming, or composite and a clear vacuum formed matrix made from a preoperative cast. For longer lasting provisionals, acrylic veneers may be made in the laboratory. Limiting the area of bonding facilitates composite removal, but the bonded area must be ground back to tooth substance when the definitive restoration is fitted. If the composite is cut without water spray it is easier to distinguish between the powdery surface of the ground composite and the glassy appearance of the underlying tooth
- Composite resin bonded to the opposing tooth to maintain occlusal contact and prevent over-eruption (eg shims or veneers where some additional occlusal reduction is required). After the definitive restoration is placed, the opposing composite is removed

• Conventional provisional restorations cemented with either a non-eugenol temporary cement or a hard cement such as zinc carboxylate. This approach may be used for adhesive restorations having some mechanical retention eg an inlay or resin bonded crown. The choice of cement will depend on how retentive the preparation is.

It is sensible to expect provisionals for adhesive preparations to be effective only in the short term. Certainly, their diagnostic usefulness in testing changes in aesthetics and occlusion is much more limited than with provisional restorations for conventional preparations.

PROBLEM SOLVING

A number of problems are encountered when making provisional restorations. Some of these are discussed below:

Insufficient bulk of material

The axial walls of resin provisionals are often thin which makes them prone to damage during removal from the mouth. This is particularly the case when minimal amounts of tooth are removed eg preparations for gold crowns. To

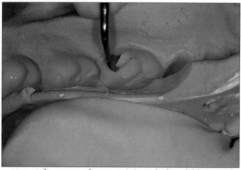

Fig. 11 Where the resulting provisional restoration would be too thin, the inside of the alginate matrix can be trimmed to give a greater bulk of resin

prevent damage, the provisional should be made temporarily wider by relieving the appropriate part of the impression with a large excavator (Fig. 11). The excess resin can be contoured after it has completely set.

Gross occlusal errors, air blows and voids

An impression matrix not being reseated fully often causes gross occlusal errors and may occur for two reasons:

• Fins of interproximal impression material being displaced and sandwiched between the impression and the occlusal surface – trim away any suspect areas from the inside of the impression with a scalpel or scissors before reseating
• Hydrostatic pressure built up within the unset resin during reseating of the impression matrix – consider cutting escape vents cut from the crown margin to the periphery of the impression with a large excavator.

Avoid voids by syringing material directly onto preparations. Of course, material is also loaded into the impression, ensuring the tip is always in the resin, to prevent the incorporation of air.

Locking in of provisional restorations

Provisional restorations are often locked in by extruded material engaging the undercuts formed by the proximal surfaces of adjacent teeth. The technique of cutting out a triangular wedge of material from the gingival embrasure space with a half Hollenback instrument has already been mentioned. This must be done while the material is still soft and before any attempt is made to remove the provisional restoration from the preparation. Once removed, any thin flash should be trimmed with a pair of scissors, and the crown reseated a number of times to ensure it does not lock into place when set.

Provisional inlays can be a particular problem because of the difficulty in removing excess resin proximally on posterior teeth. A time saving technique is possible using two light cured resins,[8] a soft one for the cavity floor and base of the box (eg Fermit), and a harder one for the occlusal surface (eg Provipont DC). A vacuum formed, transparent matrix is also needed. The softer resin is condensed into the cavity using a conventional matrix band to limit proximal extrusion. The cavity is filled to the level of the proximal contacts after which the resin surface is pock marked with a condensing instrument to provide mechanical retention for the harder resin. Following light curing the matrix band is removed. The coronal portion of the restoration is formed from the harder resin by means of the vacuum formed matrix. After light curing, the matrix is removed along with the provisional restoration, which can be further cured from the fitting surface. The amount of flash produced by this method is minimal, and the manufacturing of the inlay up to the point of trimming can be completed in less than 4 minutes.[8]

Marginal discrepancies

Although polymerisation shrinkage can cause marginal discrepancies, it is our opinion that most problems are caused simply by distortion of the margin when the provisional crown is first removed from its preparation. Such distortion results from excess material engaging proximal undercuts and can easily be prevented by following the advice in the previous section.

Should a marginal discrepancy occur with a provisional resin crown, the simplest solution is to reline it. A useful tip is to flare out the inside of the crown margin with a bur. This approach provides a greater bulk of reline material and more area for it to bond. To facilitate seating it is best not to fill the whole crown with resin, but to confine the reline material to the inner aspect of the crown margin, thus reducing hydrostatic pressure.

Multiple crowns

When several adjacent preparations require provisional restorations, reseating an impression containing resin invariably results in all the restorations being joined together as material passes through the thin and often torn interproximal

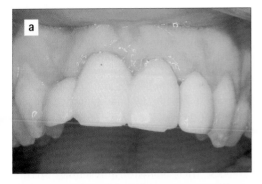

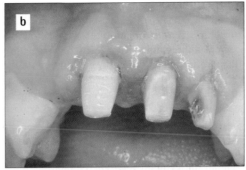

Fig. 12 Provisional restorations and gingival embrasures: (a) No gingival embrasure space provided between the maxillary incisors; (b) Bleeding from the resulting gingival inflammation prevented impressions being recorded; and (c) Patients maintain gingival health best where there are open gingival embrasures (as shown in this provisional bridge) to allow toothbrush penetration interproximally; and (d) Gingival embrasures under linked provisionals need to be opened out with a flame shaped bur

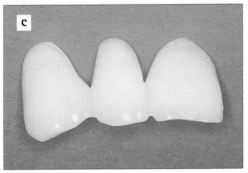

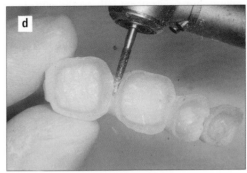

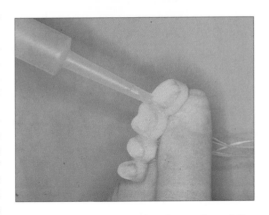

Fig. 13 A handy tip to facilitate removal of set cement (either hard or soft); loop floss under each connector of linked crowns and apply petroleum jelly to external surfaces

area. Splinting teeth together in this way has the advantage of preventing drift due to poor inter-proximal and occlusal contacts. However, it is extremely important to ensure the gingival embrasures are opened sufficiently to give good access to tooth brushing (Fig. 12a-c). This is best accomplished with a flame shaped bur (Fig. 12d).

Ideally, provisional crowns should be separate, but separation can result in unwanted gaps between them. One way[9] of overcoming this is to place small pieces of celluloid strip, roughly 1cm long, between the teeth to be prepared. The strips should have holes punched in their buccal and lingual portions with a rubber dam punch to aid retention in the over-impression. A small amount of alginate is smeared over the celluloid strip's retentive holes before seating the tray. When the impression is removed, the strips stay embedded in the alginate and separate the resin crowns while they are made.

Premature decementation

Premature loss of provisional restorations is frustrating for both patient and dentist. This problem can be largely avoided by ensuring harmony with the occlusion. A few seconds spent marking up and adjusting occlusal contacts will save time in the long run.

Occasionally, it is necessary to use a stronger cement, such as zinc polycarboxylate, especially where retention is limited.

Partial denture abutments

A provisional crown used as a partial denture abutment is made best from an acrylic resin (eg Trim) as additions are easy to make. The following technique is recommended: The provisional crown should initially be kept clear from where rest seats and guide planes are to contact. Fresh resin is then placed in these areas before reseating the partial denture with

its components lubricated with petroleum jelly. After the resin has set, the denture is removed and the crown is finished.

Eugenol containing temporary cements and adhesion

As discussed previously, eugenol-containing cements should be avoided where it is intended to cement the definitive restoration to an underlying composite core.

Removing temporary crowns

Although it is desirable for provisional crowns to remain cemented during function, they should still be easily removed when impressions are taken, adjustments are needed, or definitive restorations need cementing. When preparations are of optimal height and taper, the use of even comparatively weak temporary cements may make removal difficult, especially when the provisional restoration needs to remain undamaged for recementation or when definitive crowns are cemented on a temporary basis.

To make removal easier, the cement should be applied in a ring around the inner aspect of the margin. Alternatively, the manufacturer's

1. Wise M D. Stability of gingival crest after surgery and before anterior crown lengthening. Br Dent J 1985; 53: 20-23.
2. Crispin B J, Caputo A A. Color stability of temporary restorative materials. J Prosthet Dent 1979; 42: 27-33.
3. Moulding M B, Teplitsky P E. Intrapulpal temperature during direct fabrication of provisional restorations. Int J Prosthodont 1990; 3: 299-304.
4. Donovan T E, Hurst R G, Campagni W V. Physical properties of acrylic resin polymerized by four different techniques. J Prosthet Dent 1985; 54: 522-524.
5. Tjan A H, Castelnuovo J, Shiotsu G. Marginal fidelity of crowns fabricated from six proprietary provisional materials. J Prosthet Dent 1997; 77: 482-485.
6. Lang R, Rosentritt M, Leibrock A, Behr M, Handel G. Colour stability of provisional crown and bridge restoration materials. Br Dent J 1998; 185: 468-471.
7. Gulati A J. Physical properties of provisional restorative materials [MSc]. University of Newcastle Upon Tyne, 1996.
8. Nicholson J W, Chan D C. Two-step

provisional technique for onlay preparations. *J Esthetic Dent* 1992; **4:** 202-207.

9. Liebenberg W H. Improving interproximal access in direct provisional acrylic resin restorations. *Quintessence Int* 1994; **25:** 697-703.

10. Shillingburg H T, Hobo S, Whitsett L D. Provisional Restorations. *Fundamentals of Fixed Prosthodontics.* 4 ed pp.225-256. Chicago: Quintessence international, 1998.

11. Civjan S, Huget E F, De Simon L B. Compatibility of resin composites with varnishes, liners and bases. *J Dent Res* (Special issue) 1973; **52:** 65 (Abstract no.27).

12. Dilts W E, Miller R C, Miranda F J, Duncanson M G J. Effect of zinc oxide -eugenol on shear bond strength of selected core/cement combinations. *J Prosthet Dent* 1986; **55:** 206-208.

13. Schwartz R S, Davis R D, Mayhew R W. The effect of a ZOE temporary cement on the bond strength of a resin luting agent. *Am J Dent* 1990; **3:** 28-31.

14. Schwartz R, Davis R, Hilton T J. Effect of temporary cements on the bond strength of a resin cement. *Am J Dent* 1992; **5:** 147-150.

15. Woody T L, Davis R D. The effect of eugenol-containing and eugenol-free temporary cements on microleakage in resin bonded restorations. *Operative Dent* 1992; **17:** 175-180.

16. Millstein P L, Nathanson D. Effects of temporary cementation on permanent cement retention to composite resin cores. *J Prosthet Dent* 1992; **67:** 856-859.

modifier should be added to the cement (Fig. 5). Equal lengths of base and catalyst with a third of a length of modifier will soften the cement appreciably. Therefore, the proportion of modifier needs to be gauged for each case. Either finger pressure or instruments such as towel clips can then remove the restorations, without risking damage to the preparation margin.

Removal of excess cement

Temporary cement removal is facilitated by pre-applying petroleum jelly to the outside of the restorations and placing floss under each connector of linked crowns before seating (look at Fig. 13). Once set, the excess cement is easily removed with the strategically positioned floss.

CONCLUSION

Quality restorative dentistry needs quality provisional restorations for predictable results. Dentists therefore need to be familiar with the range of materials and techniques for short term, medium-term and long-term temporisation. Forethought and planning are also needed to ensure the most appropriate provisional is used, especially when multiple teeth are to be prepared or where occlusal or aesthetic changes are envisaged. Such changes are best tried out with provisionals so that modifications can easily be made intra-orally and when satisfactory copied into the definitive restorations. In this respect an initial diagnostic wax-up is invaluable to facilitate the construction of laboratory formed provisionals or matrices.

List of products mentioned in the text:

Fermit	Ivoclar-Vivadent UK Ltd, Leicester, UK
Protemp II (hand-mix)	ESPE, Seefeld, Germany
Protemp Garant (syringe mix)	ESPE, Seefeld, Germany
Provipont DC	Ivoclar-Vivadent UK Ltd, Leicester, UK
Quicktemp	Davis, Schottlander & Davis Ltd, Letchworth, UK
Snap	Parkell, Farmingdale, USA
Soflex Discs	3M Dental Products, St Paul, USA
Temp Bond	Kerr UK Ltd, Peterborough, UK
Temp Bond NE	Kerr UK Ltd, Peterborough, UK
Trim II	Harry J. Bosworth Co, Illinois, USA
Vita Autopolymerizing K+B Acrylics	Panadent, London, UK

- An overview of impression materials
- A rationale is put forward for the choice of elastomeric materials
- Solutions are provided to common problems encountered by the clinician in producing good, accurate impressions
- An emphasis on the need for feedback between the laboratory and the dentist

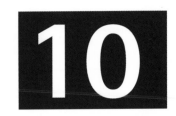

Crowns and other extra-coronal restorations: Impression materials and technique

R. W. Wassell[1] D. Barker[2] and A. W. G. Walls[3]

Well-fitting indirect restorations can only be made if there are accurate models of the oral tissues available, made from high quality impressions. Waiting for an impression to set may be more stressful for the dentist than the patient. Should the impression need to be repeated there is the embarrassment of having to explain this to the patient, the cost implications of material and time wasted and the aggravation of running late for the next appointment. Yet, if a 'Nelsonian' eye is turned to a defective impression we can only expect a substandard restoration in return.

[1]Senior Lecturer in Restorative Dentistry, [2]Higher Specialist Trainee, [3]Professor, Department of Restorative Dentistry, The Dental School, Newcastle upon Tyne NE2 4BW;
*Correspondence to: Dr R. W. Wassell, Department of Restorative Dentistry, The Dental School, Newcastle upon Tyne NE2 4BW
E-mail: R.W.Wassell@newcastle.ac.uk

Sometimes impression defects only come to light after the cast has been poured. Thus laboratory inspection is an important part of quality control, but many technicians find it difficult to feed back to their dentists for fear of the messenger being shot. Feedback between laboratory and dentist is critical to the establishment of an open and honest relationship. Hopefully, an improved understanding of impression materials coupled with techniques to overcome problems will encourage higher standards and the confidence to accept appropriate advice.

The first part of this article considers the factors influencing choice of impression material. To have a practical understanding of impression materials it is not necessary to have a PhD in dental materials science. Nevertheless, to select an appropriate material it does help to have a feel for the classification of impression materials as well as concepts such as working time, setting time, permanent deformation and dimensional stability. There are certainly other important factors that will influence your decision such as ease of manipulation, taste and tackiness but these have so far eluded quantitative measurement.

The putty-wash technique has proven popular not least for its ease of handling, but there are drawbacks that can have significant effects on its accuracy and these will be discussed.

The final part of the article will consider how to overcome the problems routinely encountered in recording impressions.

CLASSIFICATION OF IMPRESSION MATERIALS

Impression materials are commonly classified by considering their elastic properties once set. Therefore, they can be broadly divided into non-elastic and elastic materials as shown in Figure 1. Non-elastic impression materials are generally not used for obtaining impressions of crown preparations because of their inability to accurately record undercuts. The elastic impression materials can be divided into two groups: the hydrocolloids and the synthetic elastomers. Table 1. details the physical properties of the major groups of elastic impression materials available.

Hydrocolloid impression materials

The two types of hydrocolloids used in dental impressions are agar and alginate. Agar is a reversible hydrocolloid because it can pass repeatedly between highly viscous gel and low viscosity sol simply through heating and cooling. However, alginate once converted to the gel form cannot be converted back into the sol, and is therefore said to be irreversible hydrocolloid material.

Agar and alginate may be used independently or in combination to record crown impressions. Agar was first introduced into dentistry for recording crown impressions in 1937 by Sears[1] and was the first elastic impression material available. It is not commonly used in dental practice today however, because of the need for expensive conditioning baths and water cooled trays. Alginate, unlike agar, does not require any special equipment. Being easy to use and inexpensive it is popular for less critical applications eg opposing casts and study models.

Alginate and agar produce impressions with reasonable surface detail. They are both relatively hydrophilic and are not displaced from wet surfaces as easily as the elastomers.[2] However, in respect of recording crown prepara-

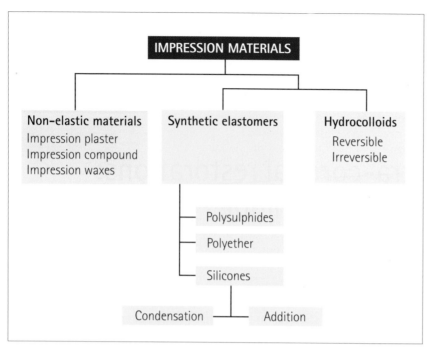

Fig. 1 Classification of impression materials

IMPRESSION MATERIALS

Non-elastic materials
Impression plaster
Impression compound
Impression waxes

Synthetic elastomers

Hydrocolloids
Reversible
Irreversible

Polysulphides

Polyether

Silicones

Condensation — Addition

tions these materials have two major disadvantages. Firstly, very poor dimensional stability because of the ready loss or imbibition of water on standing in dry or wet environments respectively. Secondly, low tear resistance which can be a real problem when attempting to record the gingival sulcus.

Some work supports the use of combined reversible and irreversible hydrocolloid impression systems.[3,4] These systems are used in a way similar to the putty-wash technique for silicone rubbers described later in this article, with the agar injected around the preparation to capture surface detail and the more viscous alginate in the impression tray. The advantages of this combination system compared with agar or alginate used individually is the minimisation of equipment required to record an agar impression (no water cooled tray is needed) and the fact that agar is more compatible with gypsum model materials than alginate. It is also relatively cheap in comparison to many synthetic elastomers. Lin et al.[5] demonstrated that the accuracy of this combination system is better than either the reversible or irreversible materials used separately and is comparable to that of polysulphide impression materials. However, the problems of low tear resistance and poor dimensional stability still apply resulting in the need for impressions to be cast up immediately. For these reasons, most practitioners tend to reject the hydrocolloids in favour of the synthetic elastomers to produce accurate and stable impressions.

The synthetic elastomers
First introduced in the late 1950s, synthetic elastomeric impression materials quickly became popular as dental materials because they significantly reduced the two main prob-

lems associated with the hydrocolloids, namely poor dimensional stability and inadequate tear resistance.

Polysulphides
The polysulphide impression materials have the longest history of use in dentistry of all the elastomers. Interestingly, they were first developed as an industrial sealant for gaps between sectional concrete structures.[6] They are available in a range of viscosities namely, light bodied (low viscosity), medium or regular bodied and heavy bodied (high viscosity).

These are now relatively unpopular materials. The setting reaction of polysulphides tends to be long with setting times often in excess of 10 minutes (acceleration is possible by adding a small drop of water to the mix). They are also messy to handle and have an objectionable odour.

Dies resulting from polysulphide impressions are generally wider and shorter than the tooth preparation. This distortion, which worsens the longer the delay in pouring up, is the result of impression shrinkage which is directed towards the impression tray — hence the wider die. Shrinkage occurs firstly as a result of a continued setting reaction after the apparent setting time, and secondly through the evaporation of water produced as a by-product of the setting reaction. A special tray, providing a 4 mm uniform space, is needed to reduce distortion from the shrinkage of a large bulk of material. The recommended maximum storage time of the set impression is about 48 hours.[6]

A significant advantage of polysulphide, however, is its long working time. This is especially useful when an impression of multiple preparations is required and some dental schools stock a few tubes to help students deal with this difficult situation. Another advantage of these materials is that they possess excellent tear resistance, undergoing considerable tensile strain before tearing. Unfortunately, their elastic properties are not ideal and some of this strain may not be recovered (high value for stress relaxation 2 minutes after setting time — see Table 1). To optimise the recovery of these viscoelastic materials, the impression should be removed with a single, swift pull as the strain imparted on the material is a function of the time for which the load is applied. This method of removal of impressions should be adopted when using any impression material, irrespective of its elastic properties.

Polyethers
A popular polyether impression material, Impregum (Espe GmbH, Germany), was the first elastomer to be developed specifically for use in dentistry and introduced in the late 1970s. Initially available only in a single 'regular' viscosity, slight modification of the viscosity is possible with the use of a diluent. More recently a heavy light bodied system has been intoduced (Permadyne, Espe GMbH, Germany).

Polyether impression materials tend to have a fast setting time of less than 5 minutes and, for this reason, have been popular for the recording of single preparations in general practice. In contrast to polysulphides, they undergo an addition cured polymerisation reaction on setting which has no reaction by-product resulting in a material with very good dimensional stability. The set material may however swell and distort because of the absorption of water on storage in conditions of high humidity. Impressions should therefore be stored dry. They should also not be stored in direct sunlight. Ideally, impressions should be poured within 48 hours of them being recorded.[6] An advantage of their relative hydrophilicity is that polyether impression materials are more forgiving of inadequate moisture control than the hydrophobic polysulphides and silicone rubbers.

Polyether impression materials have adequate tear resistance and very good elastic properties. However they do have a high elastic modulus and consequently are relatively rigid when set, hence considerable force may be required to remove the impression from both the mouth and the stone cast (Table 1, stress to give 10% compression). This may preclude their use in cases where severe undercuts are present.

Silicones
Silicone impression materials are classified according to their method of polymerisation on setting, viz. condensation curing (or Type I) silicones and addition curing (or Type II) silicones.

Silicone rubbers are available in a similar range of viscosities to the polysulphides (ie light, medium and heavy). However, the range is supplemented by a fourth viscosity; a very high viscosity or 'putty' material. The high filler loading of the putty was initially devised to reduce the effects of polymerisation shrinkage. The putty is commonly combined with a low viscosity silicone when recording impressions, a procedure known as the 'putty-wash technique' which will be discussed in some detail later in the article.

Condensation curing silicones were introduced to dentistry in the early 1960s. As with the polysulphides, the setting reaction produces a volatile by-product, but with type I silicones it is ethyl alcohol, not water. Loss of the by-product leads to measurable weight loss accompanied by shrinkage of the impression material on storage.

The dimensional changes of condensation silicones are slightly greater than those of polysulphides, but the changes in both types of material are small in comparison to the changes which occur with alginate. Nevertheless, to produce the most accurate models, regular and heavy body impressions should be cast within 6 hours of being recorded.[6] This may be a problem if the laboratory is not close to the practice.

In contrast, addition cured silicone rubbers are considered the most dimensionally stable impression materials. Like polyethers, they set, not unexpectedly, by an addition cured polymerisation reaction. No by-product is produced during cross-linkage resulting in an extremely stable impression which has been shown to remain unchanged over a substantial period of time, hence allowing impressions to be poured at leisure some days after they were recorded.

As with polysulphides, silicone rubbers are very hydrophobic so unless the teeth are properly dried 'blowholes' are likely to be produced in the set impression.

Both types of silicone rubber have the best elastic properties of any impression material, the recovery of strain being said to be almost instantaneous (Table 1, stress relaxation at 2 minutes after setting time). Like the other elastomers, they have adequate tear resistance. They are non-toxic and absolutely neutral in both colour and taste.

A great deal of recent research has been centred around the production of hydrophilic silicone rubbers. Some commercial addition cured products have recently been introduced (eg Take 1 Kerr US, Misssouri USA). A study by Pratten and Craig[7] showed one of these 'hydrophilic' addition silicone materials to have a wettability similar to that of polyethers. Other studies have also shown that treatment of impression materials with topical agents, including surfactants, results in a decrease in the number of voids found in the final impression and the dies poured from them.[8–11]

THE PROBLEMS OF PUTTY-WASH
The putty-wash technique is probably that most commonly used in general dental practice. As with most techniques it has its problems, the most common of which is invisible when the impression is recorded only becoming apparent when the restoration is tried in and fails to seat satisfactorily.

Table 1 Properties of elastomeric impression materials

Property	Polysulphides	Condensation silicones	Addition silicones	Polyethers
Coefficient of thermal expansion ($10^{-6}\,^{\circ}C^{-1}$)	270	190	190	300
Volumetric polymerisation concentration (%)	0.3	1.0	0.4	0.4
Weight Loss at 24h (%)	0.15	0.9	0.05	0.02
Stress to give 10% compression (MPa)	70	110	160	400
Stress relaxation (%) at 2 mins after setting time	45	10	5	11
Tear strength (MPa)	0.5	1.6	2.8	1.5
Elongation at break (%)	500	350	150	300

As has been mentioned already, putties were developed initially to reduce the shrinkage of condensation silicones, but the heavy filler loading is not needed for addition silicones since their polymerisation contraction and dimensional stability are in any case excellent. Presumably, addition silicone putty-wash impressions are preferred principally for their handling characteristics.

There are essentially three ways of recording a putty-wash impression:

- *One stage impression* – putty and wash are recorded simultaneously (also called twin mix or laminate technique)
- *Two stage unspaced* – putty is recorded first and after setting relined with a thin layer of wash
- *Two stage spaced* – as for two stage unspaced except a space is created for the wash. This space may be made by:
  - Polythene spacer over the teeth prior to making the putty impression
  - Recording the putty impression before tooth preparation
  - Gouging away the putty and providing escape channels for the wash.

The problem that causes invisible, but sometimes gross distortions, is recoil. Recoil can result in poorly fitting restorations and makes a mockery of using what should be accurate materials. Recoil works in the following way. Considerable forces are needed to seat putty impressions, which can result either in outward flexion of the tray wall or the incorporation of residual stresses within the material. On removing the tray from the mouth the tray walls rebound resulting in dies, which are undersized buccolingually.[12] This has been demonstrated clearly with plastic stock trays used with the one stage technique.

Although putties of lower viscosity are available they produce similar distortions with plastic trays.[13-15] Rigid metal trays however can minimise such distortions and are to be recommended for putty-wash impressions.

The two stage technique is not immune to distortion which may occur as follows:

1. Where it is used unspaced hydrostatic pressures can be generated during the seating of the wash impression, which can cause deformation and subsequent putty recoil[2] on removal. This problem can occur even with rigid trays. It may be reduced but not necessarily eliminated by spacing.
2. The putty impression may not be reseated properly causing a stepped occlusal surface of the cast and a restoration requiring excessive occlusal adjustment. It is often difficult to reseat an impression where the material has engaged undercuts especially interproximally. As such, unspaced or just locally relieved impressions are most at risk.

In summary, the most convenient and reliable way of recording a putty-wash impression is to use the one stage technique with addition silicone putty in a rigid metal tray. There is no doubt that plastic stock trays are convenient but whilst unreliable with putty-wash they can produce accurate results with a combination of heavy and light bodied addition silicones.[12-14] Special trays are only needed for heavy light bodied addition silicone impressions where stock trays are a poor fit.

DISINFECTION OF IMPRESSION MATERIALS

It has long been recognised that a potential exists for cross-infection as a result of contaminated dental impressions.[16-18] Consequently such impressions pose a hazard to laboratory personnel; it is therefore important that all impressions are disinfected prior to being transferred to a laboratory.

A study by Blair and Wassell (1996)[19] considered a number of solutions used for disinfecting impression materials. It highlighted that there is no universally recognised impression disinfection protocol available but showed that the use of a disinfectant of some description, at least in dental hospitals, had increased from 1988.[20] The recommendations of the study are supported by the British Dental Association;[21] namely that all impressions should at least undergo a disinfecting procedure by immersion in 1% sodium hypochlorite for a minimum of ten minutes.

PROBLEM SOLVING

At Newcastle senior members of staff check all impressions for indirect restorations on removal from the mouth and again in the laboratory. It is surprising how often an impression, appearing satisfactory to a cursory glance, is fatally flawed when viewed alongside the resulting cast. We would encourage dentists to audit their own work in this way with peer review providing the best stimulus for improvement.

Visible flaws related to impression technique which occur commonly include:

- Finish line not visible
- Air bubbles in critical places
- Voids or drags
- Unset impression material on surface of impression and cast

Invisible impression flaws, resulting in an apparently good fit of the restoration on the die but a poor fit on the tooth, may also occur because of:

- Tray and impression recoil (as described for the putty-wash technique)
- Detachment of impression from tray
- Permanent deformation

Where multiple preparations are recorded the likelihood of an impression defect occurring is increased and it is useful to have strategies to cope with this problem.

Whilst we cannot cover every eventuality we hope that the advice given below will help in reducing problems. Specific techniques have

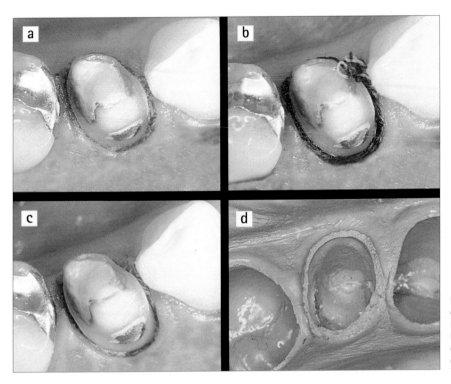

Fig. 2 Two cord technique: (a) A piece of fine retraction cord is placed in the gingival sulcus; (b) A thicker cord is placed over the first leaving a tag for removal; (c) The thicker cord is removed after washing (note clearly defined sulcus); and (d) The resulting impression of the lower first premolar

been summarised in the tables. For full accounts of potentially damaging – but useful techniques, such as electrosurgery and rotary curettage, the reader is referred elsewhere.[22]

Visible flaws
Finish line not visible
If the technician cannot identify the finish line on the impression, the resulting crown will inevitably have a poor fit with a compromised prognosis. It is therefore of some concern that recent studies report impression defects at the finish line in over a third of cases.[23,24] These defects are usually the result of inadequate gingival management in the following circumstances:

Gingival inflammation and bleeding. Every effort should be made to ensure that tooth preparations are being carried out in a healthy mouth which means patients should have effective periodontal treatment prior to recording impressions for definitive restorations. Bleeding from inflamed gingivae will displace impression material resulting in an inaccurate cast. Furthermore, if inflammation has not been controlled and a sub gingival margin placed, there is a risk of gingival recession leaving the margin as an unsightly tide line. Where the potential for a successful outcome is low, it is often sensible to delay taking the impression until the gingival condition is resolved.

Certainly there are times when contours and ledges on pre-existing defective restorations make it impossible for the patient alone to resolve the inflammation. Prior to recording the impression the defective part, or more usually the whole restoration, should be removed and a well contoured provisional restoration placed. In order to obtain a satisfactory margin on the provisional restoration some localised electro-

surgery and gingival retraction may be required (see later). Leading up to the removal of the defective restoration and during the time of temporisation, it may be helpful to prescribe an antimicrobial rinse (eg Chlorhexidine gluconate 0.12%) for 2 weeks.

Subgingival finish line. The more subgingival a preparation the more difficult it is to record the finish line adequately. Preparations finished at the gingival margin can occasionally be recorded without gingival retraction, but retraction cord will often give a more predictable result. Preparations finished within the gingival sulcus will certainly require gingival retraction. Any one or a combination of means can achieve retraction:

- Retraction cord (plain or impregnated) with or without accompanying solution
- Two-cord technique (described in Fig. 2)
- Rotary curettage
- Electrosurgery
- Copper ring

The techniques (summarised in Table 2) become potentially more invasive towards the bottom of the list but may be essential to manage more difficult cases. We find the most consistently helpful approach for subgingival impressions to be the 'two-cord' technique[25] used with ferric sulphate solution (Table 3) where necessary in combination with electrosurgery (Fig. 3). The principal advantage of the technique is that the first cord remains in place within the sulcus thus reducing the tendency of the gingival cuff to recoil and displace partially set impression material. This approach not only helps to control gingival haemorrhage and exudate but also overcomes the problem of the sulcus impression tearing because of inadequate bulk – an especially important consideration

Table 2 Techniques to capture subgingival finish lines

	Description	Indications	Comments	Hazards
Retraction cord	Standard method of retraction using twisted or knitted cord	Gingival or subgingival finish lines.	Single cord often results in inadequate gingival retraction. Two cord technique where first small diameter cord is left in place during impression recording improves definition. Wetting the cord just before removal helps control haemorrage even when solutions used (see below). Occasionally the first cord provides sufficient retraction and the second cord is not needed. Obviously, no cord tag should protrude from the sulcus whilst the impression is recorded.	Trauma and recession from excessive packing pressure. Cord contaminated by gloves may prevent impression of gingival sulcus from setting Florid inflammation if first cord not removed.
Chemical solutions	Used to soak retraction cord prior to insertion and may be applied topically to stop gingival bleeding. Solutions include: Epinephrine (1:1000 conc.) Alum (eg Aluminium potassium sulphate) Ferric Sulphate (15.5%)	Best used routinely with retraction cords — plain cords result in bleeding on removal in >50% cases.[38] Impregnated cords twice as effective if first soaked in solution.[39] With ferric sulphate the initially soaked cord can be removed from the sulcus and further solution applied with a special applicator to help stabilise the coagulum.	Alum and epinephrine similarly haemostatic,[39] retractive[40] and both give minimal postoperative inflammation.[41] Clinically, ferric sulphate appears better haemostatic agent but needs to be rubbed firmly onto bleeding gingival sulcus. Solutions need to be washed off before impression recorded.	Concerns over 'epinephrine syndrome' (raised heart rate, respiratory rate and blood pressure) when epinephrine solution used on lacerated gums in susceptible patients.[42] Concentrated solutions of Alum can cause severe inflammation and tissue necrosis.[43] Solutions will concentrate if top left off bottle. Ferric sulphate can stain the gums yellow-brown for a few days.
Electrosurgery	Controlled tissue destruction by rapid heating from radio frequency (>1.0 MHz) electrical current passing from wire tip (high current density) through patient's body into large area collecting electrode (low current density).	Uses: 1. Widen gingival sulcus (troughing) before cord placed. NB Avoid using on thin gingiva as unwanted recession can result. 2. Gingivectomy for overgrown tissue or to crown lengthening 3. Coagulation (ball electrode) but produces most tissue destruction and slow healing.	Current types: Troughing- 'cut/coag' setting (fully rectified, filtered) Gingevectomy— 'cut' setting (fully rectified) Coagulation- 'coag' setting (unrectified, damped)	Contra-indicated in patients with cardiac pacemakers.[22] Modern pacemakers are relatively well shielded[44] but still good practice to evacuate pacemaker patients from adjacent areas.To avoid unwanted arcing and tissue burns use plastic mirrors and check integrity of tip insulation. Similarly, do not touch against metal restorations. Keep collecting electrode away from rings and buckles etc.
Rotary curettage (Gingettage)	Use of chamfered diamond bur to remove epithelial tissue within healthy sulcus to expose subgingival finish line during its preparation.[45]	For subgingival preparations in healthy gingivae. Gingival sulcus depth must not exceed 3 mm and there should be adequate keratinised gingivae.[46]	Palatal tissues respond better than thinner buccal tissues..[47] Not suitable technique if a periodontal probe in the sulcus can be seen through the gingiva.	A slight deepening of the sulcus may result.[47] Poor tactile sensation during instrumentation gives high potential for overextension and damage.
Copper ring	A closely adapted copper ring is used as a vehicle to carry impression material subgingivally. A rigid impression material (composition) or an elastomer may be used.	Often used in an attempt to retrieve the situation where multiple preparations are recorded in an elastomeric impression and a localised impression defect has occurred	Dies from composition impressions are either electro formed or made in amalgam. Elastomeric copper ring impressions can also be cast in stone.	Attempts to locate a die from a copper ring impression into the relevant recess in a full arch elastomeric impression are rarely accurate and best avoided for bridgework.

with the hydrocolloids, which have low tear strength. The main disadvantage of the two-cord technique is failing to remove the first cord thereby inflicting a painful, florid gingival reaction. It is worth pointing out that where ferric sulphate solution is used, it must be applied firmly in order to stabilise the coagulum. This approach differs to the gentle technique used with other solutions.

Preparations that extend beyond the epithelial attachment may have finish lines adjacent to the alveolar bone. In such cases the above techniques are unsuitable and surgical crown lengthening with osseous recontouring may be indicated to ensure that the gingival attachment has an adequate biological width (ie 2–4 mm of gingival tissue above the alveolar crest).[26]

Brägger et al.[27] have shown that whilst in most patients the gingival margin is stable following crown lengthening, in 12% of sites 2–4 mm of recession occurred between 6 weeks and 6 months. These findings emphasise the need, in aesthetically critical areas, to delay recording the impression until the stability of the gingival margin is assured.

Localised gingival overgrowth. This annoying problem is often seen when replacing crowns with open margins where an ingrowth of inflamed gingiva prevents access to the finish line. It also occurs after a patient loses a crown with subgingival margins or a poor quality temporary crown is cemented prior to the impression stage. In these circumstances packing with retraction cord can be onerous and may be useless. A

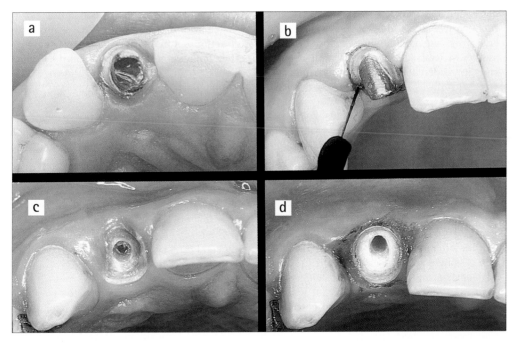

Fig. 3 'Troughing' with electrosurgery prior to packing retraction cord (a, b). The buccal tissues are relatively thin and great care is needed to avoid recession. Where subgingival finish lines need to be uncovered (c,d) electrosurgery is invaluable. Sufficient haemostasis can usually be achieved with ferric sulphate solution to allow the impression to be recorded

better approach is to remove the overgrown tissue with electrosurgery and then use a fine, straight-wire electrode to create a sulcular trough into which retraction cord may be placed (Fig. 3).

Retraction cord displaced from sulcus. In this circumstance the gingival tissues conspire to eject the cord from the sulcus almost immediately after placement. This frustration may occur where healthy gingivae are tightly bound to the tooth or where there are adjacent tooth preparations. In the latter situation placement of cord into one proximal sulcus compresses the papilla and displaces the cord already packed into the adjacent sulcus. Again, electrosurgery to create a trough into which the cord may be packed is the easiest way to deal with the problem. It is inappropriate to use electrosurgery where the gingival tissues are thin, eg buccal aspects of lower incisors, as unwanted gingival recession may result. Where the tissue is thin a small diameter retraction cord should be packed carefully using a sustained, controlled force. A half Hollenback amalgam carver or proprietary cord packing instrument is useful for the purpose. A second instrument can be used to help retain cord already packed.

Air bubbles in critical places

Air bubbles in impressions form either as a result of mixing, tray loading, syringing or tray seating. Compared with spatulation, syringe mix systems significantly reduce incorporated bubbles but are not foolproof.[28] Prior to placing the mixing nozzle, a small amount of material should be extruded from the cartridge to ensure no blockage present. A partial blockage will make extrusion difficult and detrimentally alter the base-catalyst ratio. A complete blockage can cause the cartridge to rupture. Blockages can usually be cleared with a Briault probe.

Syringing impression material around a preparation requires a certain amount of skill.

Table 3 Gingival retraction using ferric sulphate solution

- Ensure adequate isolation and moisture control – a flanged salivary ejector is needed for impressions of lower posterior teeth.
- Consider need for electrosurgery (either troughing or gingivectomy or both), one or two cord technique. If gingival inflammation needs to be resolved, temporise with well fitting margins
- Soak cord in ferric sulphate solution (15.5% w/v) and pack
- Apply further solution using syringe applicator or pledget of cotton wool (beware – solution tastes foul)
- After 5 minutes wash cord well and remove carefully so that lining of sulcus is not stripped out
- Continue to wash preparation with atomised spray and dry well, especially the more inaccessible parts of the preparation. The inner aspect of the sulcus will often appear black with stabilised coagulum. Remove any coagulum adhering to tooth preparation or finish line
- Only start mixing the impression if the gingivae are adequately retracted and dry
- If bleeding starts, reapply ferric sulphate solution and repack with soaked cord for a further 5 to 10 minutes before reattempting impression

---

Air can easily be trapped at the gingival sulcus as the syringe tip circumnavigates the tooth and a good tip is to keep the syringe tip in the expressed material during syringing. Another piece of good advice where access for the tip is restricted is to start syringing from the most difficult area – usually the disto-lingual. First express the material into the distal interproximal sulcus so that it extrudes through to the buccal. Continue along the lingual sulcus and then express material into the mesial interproximal sulcus again extruding through to the buccal. Next place the syringe tip into the disto buccal extrusion and syringe along buccally finishing with the tip in the mesial extrusion. Finally syringe up onto the occlusal surface and then use a three in one syringe to blow the light body evenly over the preparation.

Voids and drags

To obtain a void free impression it is necessary for the material to wet the teeth and soft tissues. In addition, the tray must effectively constrain the material to prevent it from flowing away from critical areas thus inducing impression drags that are commonly seen on the distal aspects of teeth adjacent to edentulous spaces and in undercut regions. Preparations and occlusal surfaces must be adequately dried with a three in one syringe or the relatively hydrophobic elastomers will be repelled and, much like a skidding lorry on a wet motorway, aquaplane away from the tooth. We have found the new generation of hydrophilic addition silicones (eg Take 1, Kerr US, Misssouri USA) to offer much improved performance in overcoming these effects.

All experienced dentists will recognise the scenario of repeating an impression only to find that the offending void or drag has reappeared in the same place. The cause is often a poorly adapted tray and the answer is to either adapt the stock tray with a rigid material (eg compound) to give more consistent spacing in the critical area or have a special tray made up. Special trays are best avoided for putty-wash impressions since there is a significant risk of the rigid, set impression locking into undercuts and then having to be cut free from the patient's mouth.

Gingival control has already been considered but it is worth re-emphasising that crevicular fluid and haemorrhage will displace impression material and result in voids and rounded, indistinct finish lines.

Yet another cause of voids is premature syringing of impression material intra-orally prior to seating the tray. The set of the syringed material is accelerated by the warmth of the mouth, resulting in a poor bond between syringed and tray materials and the appearance of a fissure at the interface between them. This type of void may be exacerbated by salivary contamination of the syringed material. The skilful use of cotton wool rolls, flanged salivary ejector and high volume aspiration is critical to effective moisture control.

Unset impression material
This problem usually does not become apparent until the impression is cast-up and a telltale smear of unset impression material is seen on the surface of the die and the surrounding teeth; the affected stone cast often has a characteristic granular appearance. Alternatively, the putty in a putty-wash impression may refuse to set. The most likely cause of both these problems is contamination of the impression by ingredients of latex rubber gloves, which poison the choroplatinic acid catalyst of addition silicones.[29,30] Not all brands of latex gloves are responsible[31] and the simple expedients are to change brands or to use non-latex gloves (eg polyethylene) for impression procedures. Where the string variety of retraction cord is used, twisting it tight in gloved hands to make it more easily packable also has the potential to contaminate and prevent impression setting.[32] This is less of a problem with knitted or woven cords, which should not be twisted prior to insertion. Perhaps surprisingly, retraction solutions have not been shown to effect impression setting significantly.[32]

Invisible flaws
Impression and tray recoil
A visible impression flaw may be made invisible by attempting a localised reline with a little light bodied material. It may be tempting but is not good practice; seating pressures can result in impression recoil and significant distortion.[33] Moreover, the addition may bond poorly and subsequently peel away. If an impression is unsatisfactory it should be retaken.

As already discussed the use of putty-wash in non-rigid trays can result in tray wall recoil and undersized dies.

Detachment of impression from tray
Detachment of the impression from the tray can result in gross distortion of the cast. It may occur on removal from the mouth and may often go unnoticed. Prevention of detachment relies on the proper use of adhesive and having a tray with adequate perforations.[34] It is a good idea to select the tray and apply adhesive before the tooth is prepared. Doing so will allow time for the adhesive's solvent to evaporate and for adequate bond strength to develop.[35] Painting the tray immediately before recording the impression is not a good idea. This advice applies to elastomers and alginates. Alginates are more easily debonded from the tray so it is good practice to use a scalpel to cut away excess alginate from the tray heels to facilitate inspection of this vulnerable area. The excess needs to be removed before putting the impression down or the impression will distort.

Elastomeric impressions may require to be poured up more than once, especially if critical air blows in the stone affect the resulting die. The repour will be grossly inaccurate if impression material has lifted away from the tray because of the lack of adhesive.[36]

Where a special tray is made it is important that the wax spacer does not come into contact with the tray acrylic; contamination will reduce the strength of the adhesive bond. Technicians may need to be instructed to place a layer of aluminium foil over the surface of the wax before forming the tray.[35] Furthermore, a self cured acrylic tray should be made at least a day in advance to allow for its polymerisation contraction.

Permanent deformation
Withdrawal from an undercut will test an impression's elastic recovery. As already mentioned the addition silicones have good resistance to permanent deformation, however, there are situations where an impression can be deformed and the small but significant deformation is unlikely to be detected. In this respect gingival embrasure spaces cause especial difficulty in two situations. Firstly, significant gin-

gival recession with the loss of the interproximal papilla will lock set impression material into the space. The impression will either be torn on removal from the mouth or deformed or both. This problem is best dealt with by blocking out embrasure spaces with soft red wax or a proprietary blocking out material. Secondly, where there is a significant triangular interproximal space below the preparation finish line it is best to extend the finish line gingivally. The space is thereby opened up to allow the impression to be withdrawn without tearing or distortion.

Special trays should be given sufficient spacing (at least two layers of baseplate wax) to give sufficient thickness of impression material to resist undue stress and strain on removal from undercut areas.

Finally, the elastic properties of materials are not fully developed at manufacturers' stated setting times. So it is worth remembering that a significant improvement in resistance to permanent deformation occurs if addition silicone impressions are left a further minute or two before removal from the mouth.[13]

The problem of recording multiple preparations

It is always distressing when in an attempt to record multiple preparations one or two areas of the impression have a critical defect. There are several strategies for dealing with the situation:

- Retake the whole impression
- Record a separate impression of the preparation (or preparations) having the impression defect. A copper ring may be used as described previously in Table 2. The resulting die is then located in the defective region of the first impression before pouring up the master die. Not surprisingly, it can be difficult to locate the die reliably and there is a risk of causing occlusal or proximal contact discrepancies.
- Retake sufficient impressions to ensure that there is an adequate impression available of each preparation. The patient is re-appointed for a *transfer coping pick-up impression*.[37] In the interim individual dies are made by copper or silver plating (Table 4). On each die is formed an accurately fitting acrylic (Duralay, Reliance Dental Co, Illinois, USA) transfer coping. At the next appointment the transfer copings are tried onto the preparations and the fit checked. Copings having the same path of insertion are linked together with wire and

acrylic so that stability of coping position is ensured within the pick-up impression. Alternatively, excrescences of acrylic can be added to a coping to ensure it is retained within the pick-up impression. After recording the pick-up impression individual dies can be secured within their copings using sticky wax before the master cast is poured. The technique can be used with stone dies, but there is a risk of the die being abraded by the construction of the acrylic coping. This problem can be overcome by double pouring each die. The coping is made on one die, which is then discarded, and the other die is used for the master cast.

Where it is clearly going to be a problem to record many preparations on a single impression this should be taken into account and planned for. There are few cases that cannot be broken down into smaller more manageable stages even if this means using provisional restorations to stabilise the occlusion while say four or six definitive anterior crowns are constructed. When it is absolutely necessary to record simultaneously more than six teeth in one arch it is wise to use the transfer coping and pick-up impression technique from the outset.

CONCLUSION

The ability to record consistently good impressions is both a science and an art. We hope this article has shed light on both aspects. It is worth bearing in mind that the impression influences not only the quality of the subsequent restoration but also the technician's perception of the dentist's skill. As none of us can achieve perfection every time there is much to be said for encouraging technicians to feed back when they receive a substandard impression.

1. Sears A W. Hydrocolloid impression technique for inlays and fixed bridges. *Dent Digest* 1937; **43:** 230-234.
2. Brown D. An update on elastomeric impression materials. *Br Dent J* 1981; **150:** 35-40.
3. Heisler W H, Tjan A H L. Accuracy and bond strength of reversible with irreversible hydrocolloid impression systems: a comparative study. *J Prosthet Dent* 1992; **68:** 578-584.
4. Appleby D C, Parneijer C H, Boffa J. The combined reversible hydrocolloid/ irreversible hydrocolloid impression system. *J Prosthet Dent* 1980; **44:** 27-35.
5. Lin C, Zeiber G J. Accuracy of impression materials for complete arch fixed partial dentures. *J Prosthet Dent* 1988; **59:** 288-291.
6. Craig R G. *Restorative Dental Materials.* 10th ed.pp.281-332. London: Mosby, 1997.
7. Pratten D H, Craig R G. Wettability of a hydrophilic addition silicone impression material. *J Prosthet Dent* 1989; **61:** 197-202.
8. Vassilakos N, Fernandes C P, Nilner K. Effect of plasma treatment on the wettability of elastomeric impression materials. *J Prosthet Dent* 1993; **70:** 165-171.
9. Millar B J, Dunne S M, Robinson P B. The effect of a surface wetting agent on void formation in impressions. *J Prosthet Dent* 1997; **77:** 54-56.
10. Ozden N, Ayhan H, Erkut S, Can G, Piskin E. Coating of silicone-based impression materials in a glow-discharge system by acrylic acid plasma. *Dent Mat* 1997; **13:** 174-178.
11. Boening K W, Walter M H, Schuette U. Clinical significance of surface activation of silicone impression materials. *J Dent* 1998; **26:** 447-452.
12. Wassell R W, Ibbetson R J. The accuracy of polyvinylsiloxane impressions made with standard and reinforced stock trays. *J Prosthet Dent* 1991; **65:** 748-757.

Table 4 Copper and silver-plated dies; which impression materials can be electroplated

	Copper plate	Silver plate
Addition silicone	Yes	Yes
Condensation silicone	No	Some
Polyether	No	Yes
Polysulphide	No	Yes
Impression compound	Yes	No

13. Abuasi H. *Accuracy of polyvinyl siloxane impressions.* [PhD]. University of Newcastle upon Tyne, 1993.

14. Abuasi H A, Wassell R W. Comparison of a range of addition silicone putty-wash impression materials used in the one-stage technique. *Eur J Prosthodont Restor Dent* 1994; **65:** 748-757.

15. Carrotte P V, Johnson A, Winstanley R B. The influence of the impression tray on the accuracy of impressions for crown and bridgework. *Br Dent J* 1998; **185:** 580-585.

16. Ray K C, Fuller M L. Isolation of Mycobacterium from dental impression material. *J Prosthet Dent* 1963; **13:** 390-396.

17. Leung R L, Schonfeld S E. Gypsum casts as a potential source of microbial cross-contamination. *J Prosthet Dent* 1983; **49:** 210-211.

18. Powell G L, Runnells R D, Saxon B A, Whisenant B K. The presence and identification of organisms transmitted to dental laboratories. *J Prosthet Dent* 1990; **64:** 235-237.

19. Blair F M, Wassell R W. A survey of the methods of disinfection of dental impressions used in dental hopitals in the United Kingdom. *Br Dent J* 1996; **180:** 369-375.

20. Watkinson A C. Disinfection of impressions in UK dental schools. *Br Dent J* 1988; **164:** 22-23.

21. BDA. *Advice sheet A12: Infection Control in Dentistry.* pp12: British Dental Association Advisory Service, 1996.

22. Shillingburg H T, Hobo S, Whitsett L D, Jacobi R, Brackett S E. *Fundamentals of fixed prosthodontics.* 3rd ed. pp257-279. Chicago: Quintessence, 1997.

23. Carrotte P V, Winstanley R V, Green J A. A study of the quality of impressions for anterior crowns received at a commercial laboratory. *Br Dent J* 1993; **174:** 235-240.

24. Winstanley R B, Carrotte P V, Johnson A. The quality of impressions for crowns and bridges received at commercial dental laboratories. *Br Dent J* 1997; **183:** 209-213.

25. Cloyd S, Puri S. Using the double cord packing technique of tissue retraction for making crown impressions. *Dent Today* 1999; **18:** 54-59.

26. Ingber F J S, Rose L F, Coslet J G. The 'Biologic Width' - A concept in periodontics and restorative dentistry. *Alpha-Omegan* 1977; **10:** 62-65.

27. Brägger U, Lauchenauer D, Lang NP. Surgical lengthening of the clinical crown. *J Clin Periodont* 1992; **19:** 58-63.

28. Chong Y H, Soh G, Lim K C, Teo C S. Porosities in five automixed addition silicone elastomers. *Operative Dent* 1991; **16:** 96-100.

29. Noonan J E, Goldfogel M H, Lambert R L. Inhibited set of the surface of addition silicones in contact with rubber dam. *Operative Dent* 1985; **10:** 46-48.

30. Kahn R, Donovan T, Chee W. Interaction of latex gloves and polyvinylsiloxane impression materials: a screening survey. *Int J Prosthodont* 1989; **2:** 342-346.

31. Baumann M A. The influence of dental gloves on the setting of impression materials. *Br Dent J* 1995; **179:** 130-135.

32. de Camargo L M, Chee W W L, Donovan T E. Inhibition of polymerization of polyvinyl siloxanes by medicaments used on gingival retraction cords. *J Prosthet Dent* 1993; **70:** 114-117.

33. Bomberg T A, Hatch R A. Correction of defective impression by selective addition of impression material. *J Prosthet Dent* 1984; **52:** 38-40.

34. MacSween R. Peel bond strengths of five impression material tray adhesives. *J Can Dent Assoc* 1991; **57:** 654-657.

35. Davis G B, Moser J B, Brinsden G I. The bonding properties of elastomer tray adhesives. *J Prosthet Dent* 1976; **36:** 278-285.

36. Tjan A H. Comparing effects of tray treatment on the accuracy of dies. *J Prosthet Dent* 1987; **58:** 175-178.

37. Howat A P, Capp N J, Barrett N V J. *A colour atlas of occlusion & malocclusion.* pp182. Aylesbury: Wolfe Publishing Ltd, 1991.

38. Pelzner R B, Kempler D, Stark M M, Lum L B, Nicholson R J, Soelberg K B. Human blood pressure and pulse rate response to r-epinephrine retraction cord. *J Prosthet Dent* 1978; **39:** 287-292.

39. Weir D J, Williams B H. Clinical effectiveness of mechanical-chemical tissue displacement methods. *J Prosthet Dent* 1984; **51:** 326-329.

40. Bowles W H, Tardy S J, Vahadi A. Evaluation of new gingival retraction agents. *J Dent Res* 1991; **70:** 1447-1449.

41. de Gennaro G G, Landesman H M, Calhoun J E, Martinoff J T. A comparison of gingival inflammation related to retraction cords. *J Prosthet Dent* 1982; **47:** 384-386.

42. Donovan T E, Gandara B K, Nemetz H. Review and survey of medicaments used with gingival retraction cords. *J Prosthet Dent* 1985; **53:** 525-531.

43. Shaw D H, Krejci R F, Cohen D M. Retraction cords with aluminium chloride: effect on the gingiva. *Operative Dent* 1980; **5:** 138-141.

44. Riordan A T, Fosko S W. Electrosurgery and cardiac devices. *J Am Acad Dermatol* 1997; **37:** 250-255.

45. Ingraham R, Sochat R. Rotary gingival curretage – A technique for tooth preparation and management of the gingival sulcus for impression taking. *Int J Periodontol Restorative Dent* 1981; **1:** 9-33.

46. Brady W F. Periodontal and restorative considerations in rotary curettage. *J Am Dent Assoc* 1982; **105:** 231-236.

47. Kamansky F W, Tempel T R, Post A C. Gingival tissue response to rotary gingival curretage. *J Prosthet Dent* 1984; **52:** 380-383.

IN BRIEF

The stages of fitting and cementation of crowns are considered including:
- The clinical stages of try-in and adjustment of restorations prior to cementation
- Conventional and adhesive cements
- A rationale for the use of different cements based on their various physical and chemical properties
- Crown cementation with conventional cements

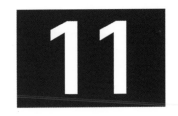

Crowns and other extra-coronal restorations: Try-in and cementation of crowns

R. W. Wassell[1] D. Barker[2] and J. G. Steele[3]

Having successfully negotiated the planning, preparation, impression and prescription of your crown, the cementation stage represents the culmination of all your efforts. This stage is not difficult, but a successful outcome needs as much care as the preceding stages. Once a restoration is cemented there is no scope for modification or repeat. You have to get it right first time. Decemented crowns often have thick layers of residual cement suggesting problems with either initial seating or cement handling. When the fate of restorations costing hundreds of pounds depends on correct proportioning of cements and the quality of the mix, the value of a well-trained and experienced dental nurse is easy to see. Both dentist and nurse need a working knowledge of the materials they are handling.

[1,3]Senior Lecturer in Restorative Dentistry, [2]Higher Specialist Trainee, Department of Restorative Dentistry, The Dental School, Newcastle upon Tyne NE2 4BW; *Correspondence to: Dr R. W. Wassell, Department of Restorative Dentistry, The Dental School, Newcastle upon Tyne NE2 4BW
E-mail: R.W.Wassell@newcastle.ac.uk

Crown seating relies on a satisfactory try-in and this subject will be covered first. We will then consider the topics of cements, their selection and usage.

TRY-IN PROCEDURE FOR CROWNS

This involves three stages: firstly pre-operative evaluation of crown on its die, secondly seating on the tooth and finally evaluation of the seated crown.

Checking the crown on the die

It is always worth checking the fit of the crown on the cast before trying it in the patient. In this way problems involving marginal fit, aesthetics and articulation can be anticipated prior to try in. Always check the fit surface of the crown for defects and the die for damage, preferably with a good light and under magnification (Table 1). Detecting these problems before try-in will allow you either to address the problem yourself or to negotiate with your laboratory from a position of strength. It is surprising how often clear ledges or deficiencies can be detected at this stage. Subsequent stages then rely on the crown being checked in the mouth and then often back on the die again when there is a problem with the fit.

Seating the crown

Having checked the crown on the cast, any temporary restoration is removed and the preparation is carefully cleaned of all residues of temporary cement, especially in retention grooves. The try-in procedure can normally (though not always) be accomplished without the need for local anaesthetic. This is advantageous in that

the patient's tactile sense is not impaired which is valuable in assessing the occlusion and tightness of proximal contacts.

The crown should be tried in without forcing it onto its preparation; if it fails to seat there are a range of reasons why this may have happened. It pays to use a systematic approach to localise problems:

1. First, ensure there is no retained temporary cement or trapped gingival tissue
2. Then check and adjust tight proximal contacts (see following section) as these often prevent seating. Also check the original cast for damage to the stone in these contact areas
3. Then re-check the crown for the most obvious laboratory errors, including casting blebs, damaged or chipped dies or grossly overextended margins. Casting blebs can be removed with a bur. Over-extended margins should be adjusted from the axial surface, not from underneath (Soflex discs are useful for this purpose – see Fig. 1). To avoid the abrasive dragging metal over the margin, run the disc so that the abrasive travels in the direction of the occlusal surface, not towards the margin
4. Where the crown still does not seat burnish marks on the internal walls of a sandblasted metal crown may indicate where it is binding. The identification of these points may be aided by the use of disclosing wax or aerosol sprays. Any imperfections may be lightly ground with a bur or stone before retrying the crown.

With modern day addition silicones, impression distortion is an unusual cause of ill-fitting restorations but may be responsible where no apparent fault can be detected on restoration or

Table 1. Check list of laboratory errors affecting marginal fit

Error	Cause	Remedy
Tight proximal contacts	Imprecise die location or abrasion of the adjacent stone contact points	Check for displacement of the dies when the crown is seated on the working cast. Identify tight contact by interposing articulating paper, grind and polish
Casting blebs on fit surface	Air bubbles trapped during investment	Identify under magnification and remove with small round bur
Over-extended crown margins	Poor impression, poor die trimming, surplus untrimmed wax or porcelain	Trim from axial surface (Fig. 1) and polish — consider returning crown to lab
Under-extended crown margins	Poor impression, poor die trimming, difficulty identifying finish line	If under-extension obvious and impression satisfactory have crown remade. Alternatively retake impression
Damaged dies	Finish line chipped because of careless handling or abraded when casting reseated with blebs or overextended margins	Always try and determine why the die is damaged. If the crown does not fit after adjusting blebs or over-extended margins return it to laboratory
No die spacer (Space needed to accommodate cement lute)	Technician not aware of technique or forgot to apply	Lack of spacer results in a tightly fitting crown which may not seat during try in and may 'lift' further after cementation

die. Problems can occur where an impression is removed too soon or where unset impression material results from glove contamination (look out for the tell tale smear of unset impression material on the surface of the cast). If you cannot get the crown to seat easily and can find no obvious reason, you may rightly suspect that there is an impression distortion. In that case, save time and just take a new one.

Finally, it is important to distinguish between a crown that rocks on its preparation because of binding somewhere on the fit surface and one that just has a loose fit resulting from the use of die spacer. In fact, tightly fitting crowns confer no additional retention after cementation[1] and may interfere with seating.

Assessment of the seated crown

There is no point in making a detailed assessment of proximal contacts, marginal fit, aesthetics and occlusion until the crown is seated fully.

Once you have got to this stage, providing you and the laboratory have taken care with preceding clinical and technical stages, minimal or no adjustment should be necessary. Again it is important to adopt a systematic approach.

Proximal contacts

The tightness of proximal contacts can be tested with dental floss and should offer some resistance but not make its passage too difficult. If these are too tight they can be ground a little at a time and polished. This requires the greatest care as it is easy to open the contact accidentally, and it is very problematic trying to rebuild it at this stage. Prior to adjustment it may be helpful to mark the proximal contact by sandwiching a small piece of articulating paper between crown and tooth either on the cast or in the mouth.

Open contact points occur less frequently and can only be modified by returning the

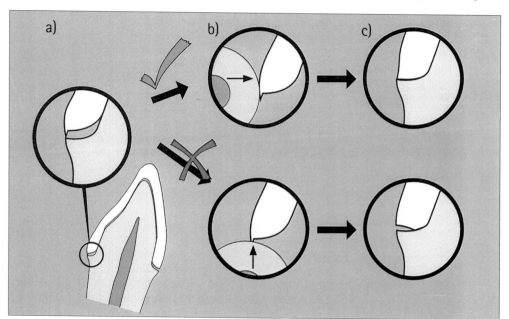

Fig. 1a) Marginal discrepancy caused by an overextended lingual margin; b) Reduce the overextension from the axial surface not from underneath; and c) Seating achieved with the axial bulk removed, incorrect adjustment results in a deficient margin

crown to the laboratory for addition of porcelain or gold solder.

Assessment of marginal fit

Crowns really must have an accurate marginal fit if you intend them to survive in the long term. There is a full spectrum of fit, from perfection (which is probably rarely achieved) to open margins around the entire crown. It is up to you, your own clinical standards and perhaps your patient at what point on that spectrum you decide that the marginal fit becomes unacceptable. A combination of clinical experience and empirical data suggest a marginal opening of 100 μm^2 is at the borderline of acceptability, especially where the margin can only be probed.[3] Maintaining the highest possible clinical standards at this stage has long-term benefits; ill-fitting margins will render the tooth more susceptible to cement dissolution, plaque retention and recurrent caries. Defective subgingival margins compromise gingival health by an alteration in local bacteria.[4]

Poor fit can present as a gap or an overhanging margin (positive ledge) or deficient margin (negative ledge). Overextended margins and positive ledges may be corrected by adjusting the crown from its axial surface until it is possible to pass a probe from tooth to crown without it catching. A larger problem, necessitating that the crown be remade if it is unacceptable, occurs when a margin remains deficient or has a negative ledge.

Gold restorations should have their accessible margins burnished before cementation. The set cement is likely to be cracked if the margin is burnished afterwards. There is no evidence that burnishing improves longevity but it can insure that a discerning patient does not catch a fingernail at the margin! The procedure involves dragging the gold from restoration to tooth using a rotary instrument such as a green stone or steel finishing bur. Where only minimal burnishing is needed a sharp hand instrument such as a proprietary gold knife or half Hollenback instrument is useful. Once burnished the restoration must be re-polished taking care to avoid the fine edge of marginal gold.

Aesthetics

For porcelain crowns, some adjustment of shape and shade is possible at this stage but it is best to ensure minimal adjustment by following the advice given in Part 6 of the series.

Grinding with diamond burs can alter crown contours and porcelain additions can be made to metal ceramic crowns if necessary. Shades that are slightly too light may be darkened by the addition of stain and re-firing while all ceramic crowns with no cores may have their shade modified slightly by the luting composite in the same way as veneers. If you anticipate the need for substantial adjustments, a try-in at biscuit bake can be specified so that the crown can be glazed when you are happy with the final appearance. Obviously the patient will need to

see the restoration and comment on it prior to cementation. If the shape and shade are clearly unacceptable it is better to acknowledge this rather than risk a dissatisfied patient with the possibility of having to cut off the restoration and repeat all the preceding stages.

Assessment of the occlusion

The occlusion is the last assessment to make, but there is no point thinking about making any adjustment to the occlusal surface until the crown is finally seated. It is then best to remove it and identify a pair of adjacent occluding teeth, termed index teeth, which, after re-seating, can be used to assess visually, and with shim stock, how much adjustment is needed.

Visually checking the occlusion gives only a gross indication of the amount of adjustment needed; articulating foils and shim stock are needed too. Figure 2 shows shim stock, which is a 10 μm thick Mylar film, held in mosquito forceps and used as a feeler gauge between occluding teeth. Shim stock can be bought from dental suppliers or can be made, very inexpensively, in the dental surgery by passing a 'space blanket' (the sort of thing marathon runners wrap around themselves after a race, available at camping shops) through an office shredder and then cutting it into 2 cm lengths.

Miller's forceps, used to support articulating

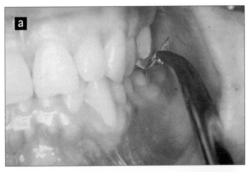
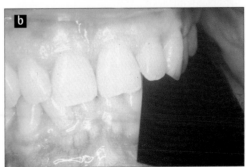
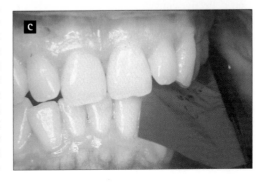
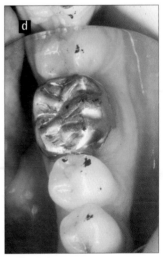

Fig. 2 Occlusal assessment. With the restoration out select a pair of index teeth, which hold shim stock (a). Mark with black articulating foil and adjust ICP (b). Mark with red and adjust excursive interferences and deflections (c). Adjustment complete (d)

foils so that they do not crumple during intra-oral placement, are also an advantage (again look at Fig. 2). Some articulating papers resemble blotting paper in consistency and thickness. They are prone to leave false marks and may alter the patient's position of closure. These papers can be as thick as 200 µm, which is over ten times as thick as the best thin foils such as GHM (GHM Occlusion Prüf Folie, Germany),[5] which are infinitely preferable. Despite their slightly higher cost, the accuracy and precision with which they will mark a restoration can save a great deal of time and effort provided the teeth are dry.

With posterior teeth, both restoration and adjacent teeth should hold shim stock firmly in the intercuspal position (ICP). With anteriors, if the other incisors hold shim stock lightly the restoration should be made to do so too. Failure to do so can result in the crowned tooth being overloaded, which in turn can cause pain, mobility, fracture or displacement. As well as using shim stock and articulating foils, it is also worth listening to the occlusion with and without the crown in place as small occlusal discrepancies can readily be heard with the teeth being tapped together.

Dentists will often have a favourite bur for occlusal adjustment. We prefer a large flame shaped diamond in an air rotor or speed increasing handpiece. Occasionally, it may be necessary to adjust the tooth opposing a restoration to avoid crown perforation or exposure of rough opaque porcelain. Such adjustments should be planned with the patient's consent and not sprung on them part way through the procedure. A thickness gauge (eg Svensen Gauge) is invaluable for predicting areas vulnerable to perforation.

Once ICP has been re-established the excursions can be checked, preferably with a different coloured foil (eg red). ICP contacts are then re-marked with the original colour (eg black) allowing the excursive contact to be differentiated and refined. The decision about whether the restoration is to be involved in guiding jaw movement (which it often is with anterior teeth) or whether there should be disclusion (as often occurs posteriorly) should have been made well before this stage and it is important you have a clear idea of the pattern of occlusal contact you are trying to achieve. Finally, it is worth guiding back the mandible into the retruded path of closure to ensure the restoration is not introducing a new deflective contact.

Occasionally, a restoration will be short of occlusion. This is used as a deliberate ploy in some laboratories to eliminate the clinical need for occlusal adjustment. A thin card spacer placed over the cast of the opposing tooth creates clearance. This may seem an innocuous, perhaps even a desirable practice, but can result in serious immediate problems presenting where multiple restorations are fitted. The lack of contacts can affect occlusal stability whilst destructive interferences may occur as teeth

erupt back into occlusion. It may often be acceptable to monitor infra-occluding restorations and adjust interferences as necessary. In more critical cases occlusal additions of porcelain or solder may be indicated or the restoration remade. The point is that it should not be necessary to do this at all because all of these problems can be avoided by taking care at the preceding stages, especially with impressions (including opposing impressions), jaw registration and temporary restorations.

Finishing and polishing
The final stage prior to cementation is polishing. A rough surface, especially in porcelain, will rapidly wear the opposing tooth[6] and so it is very important to use a sequence of abrasives designed for the material in question to achieve a smooth surface. Details of the materials we use are shown at the end of the article. Metal surfaces can be finished with finishing burs followed by rubber abrasive points (Kenda: blue, brown and green). Abrasive discs (eg Soflex) are useful for flat areas such as proximal contact points and can be used on either metal or porcelain. Porcelain can be also be finished with composite finishing diamonds (Premier: yellow and white stripe), but a light touch and water spray is needed to avoid stripping off the diamond coating. Further finishing is achieved with rubber abrasive points (Kenda: white) followed by a felt wheel or rubber cup charged with diamond polishing paste (Super Diglaze). Alternatively, a metal ceramic crown can be reglazed.

CEMENTS
When the fit of the crown is considered satisfactory and all adjustments have been made, the crown can be cemented using one of the materials described in this section.

Cements may be classified as soft or hard. Soft cements can be used for provisional cementation of definitive crowns when a trial assessment period is needed, for example if the occlusion or aesthetics is being significantly altered. Hard cements are used for definitive cementation. This article deals principally with hard cements.

Hard cements
Many types of hard cement have been developed and continue to be available. This diversity of choice suggests no one cement meets all of the requirements of an 'ideal cement' however some are more suitable than others for certain applications.

There are essentially three types of hard cement: conventional, resin or a hybrid of the two. Conventional cements (eg zinc phosphate, zinc polycarboxylate and glass ionomer) rely on an acid-base reaction resulting in the formation of an insoluble salt (the cement) and water. Resin cements set by polymerisation.

The mechanisms by which cements secure restoration to prepared tooth include non-adhesive luting, micro-mechanical bonding and molecular adhesion. The mechanisms of non-adhesive luting and micro-mechanical retention are the main methods of action of conventional cements. Molecular adhesion on the other hand is more significant in the case of resin cements and hybrid cements. Although some conventional cements have adhesive properties, such as zinc polycarboxylate and GIC, these are limited by the cement's tensile strength. Furthermore, adhesion to noble metals is negligible but can be improved in the case of GICs by the use of tin-plating. Texturing the fitting surface of the crown, as after sandblasting, increases the resistance of the cement to dynamic lateral loading.[7]

We will now go on to discuss the advantages and disadvantages of each of the major groups of cements and make recommendations for their use.

Zinc phosphate cement

Advantages
- Long track record
- Good compressive strength (if correctly proportioned)
- Good film thickness
- Reasonable working time
- Resistant to water dissolution
- No adverse effect on pulp although initially acidic

Disadvantages
- Low tensile strength
- No chemical bonding
- Not resistant to acid dissolution

Recommendations
- Good default cement for conventional crowns and posts with retentive preparations
- Working time can be extended for cementation of multiple restorations by incremental mixing and cooled slab

Zinc phosphate has the longest track record and has remained popular for luting purposes due mainly to its high compressive strength, relatively long working time and ability to form a low film thickness between crown and tooth. Look at Table 2 for the relative physical properties of cements and it is clear that in common with the other conventional cements, zinc phosphate possesses high compressive strength but

low tensile strength. It is this low tensile strength, which dictates the importance of preparation geometry in reducing the development of disruptive tensile stresses within the cement lute resulting in loss of retention of the restoration.

The retaining action of zinc phosphate cement is one of micromechanical interlocking between surface irregularities of the crown and tooth. It does not bond to tooth substance or crown material.

It is normally supplied as a powder (essentially zinc oxide) and liquid (phosphoric acid buffered with zinc and aluminium ions), which are mixed together by hand. The proportions of powder and liquid are not normally measured and therefore care must be taken to produce a 'mix', which provides a cement of low initial viscosity to form a thin film, but with sufficient powder incorporated to give adequate strength once set.[8] The powder should be incorporated in increments to prevent the cement setting too quickly as a result of the exothermic reaction. A slab cooled in the refrigerator can further extend working time. The consistency of zinc phosphate may be checked by lifting the cement on the spatula and holding it over the slab. It should string out slightly between the spatula and slab before running back onto the slab. If it requires to be pushed off the spatula it is too thick and conversely, if it runs off too quickly it is not thick enough. Given how critical this is, it is worth making sure that you and your chair side assistant both understand fully what is required, and are prepared to stop and mix again if a problem arises.

All cements are to some extent soluble. Zinc phosphate has a low solubility in water but erosion leading to loss of the cement lute and failure of the restoration is not normally associated with this cement, crowns tending to be lost more because of a poor retentive design of the preparation. However, cement erosion is seen in patients with acid regurgitation (Fig. 3).

Historically, zinc phosphate cements have been identified as having a potential irritant effect on the pulp.[9] This has been attributed to the low pH of the cement at the time of cementa-

Cement	Compressive strength (MPa)	Tensile strength (MPa)	Bond strength to dentine (MPa)	Film thickness (µm)	Solubility in water (% in 24h)	Setting time at 37°C and 100% humidity (mins)
Zinc phosphate	96–133	3.1–4.5	0	25 max	0.2 max	5–9
Zinc polycarboxylate	57–99	3.6–6.3	2.1	25–48	< 0.05	7–9
GIC	93–226	4.2–5.3	3–5	22–24	0.4–1.5	6–8
RMGI	85–126	13–24 without DBA 14–20 with DBA	10–12	10–22	0.07–0.4	5.5–6.0
Resin cement	180–265	34–37	18–30	13–20 with DBA	0.13	4–5

Table 2 Cement properties

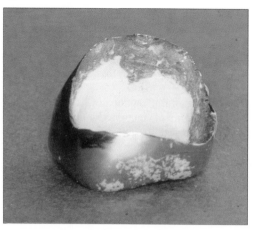

Fig. 3 Erosion of zinc phosphate cement seen in a patient with acid reflux

tion, but preparation trauma, temporisation and bacterial contamination may also have been responsible. Although zinc phosphate is acidic on mixing (pH 2–3.5 depending on brand) this acidity reduces over the first 24 hours and stabilises at a near neutral pH of 6.5. Despite this acidity Brannstrom and Nyborg[10,11] found no irritating effect on the pulp *per se* and, in practice, this potential irritant effect does not seem to be significant.

At one time cavity varnish was advocated to coat a preparation prior to cementation to protect it from cement but this adversely affected retention.[12,13] Nowadays a dentine-bonding agent could be used and, anecdotally, this has helped with some teeth, which have been sensitive after preparation, but controlled studies are needed to assess the long-term consequences. If the dentine is to be etched it is essential that the primer seals all the open tubules or sensitivity may worsen and bacterial invasion may jeopardise the pulp.

Zinc oxide eugenol cements

Cements based on zinc oxide and eugenol are classical soft cements. Attempts have been made to create a more permanent cement by adding o-ethoxy-benzoic acid (EBA) to zinc oxide-eugenol and by reinforcing it with aluminium oxide and polymethylmethacrylate. Based on *in vitro* tests, this type of cement was reported to have good strength and be less soluble than zinc phosphate cement.[14,15] Unfortunately, its performance was much poorer *in vivo* and studies have shown that it deteriorates much more rapidly in the mouth than other cements.[16,17] It cannot be recommended as a definitive lute for restorations.

Polycarboxylate cements
Advantages
- Reasonable track record
- Good compressive strength (if correctly proportioned)
- Adequate working time
- Bonds to enamel and dentine
- Adequate resistance to water dissolution (but less good than zinc phosphate)
- No adverse effect on pulp and less acidic than zinc phosphate on mixing

Disadvantages
- Low tensile strength
- Can deform under loading
- Can be difficult to obtain low film thickness
- Not resistant to acid dissolution
Recommendations
- Traditionally used for vital or sensitive teeth, but no evidence to support efficacy (dentine bonding agents used to seal preparation prior to cementation may be a better option)
- Occasionally useful to retain an unretentive provisional crown

Zinc polycarboxylate (or zinc polyacrylate) has a relatively long history as a luting cement. Unlike zinc phosphate, polycarboxylate cement does bond to tooth tissue, its bond strength to enamel being greater than that to dentine. It also bonds to stainless steel so dental instruments must be cleaned before the material sets to prevent a tenacious bond forming.

The tensile strength of polycarboxylate compares favourably to that of zinc phosphate although its compressive strength tends to be lower and it is difficult to achieve an equally low film thickness.

Zinc polycarboxylate cement is not as acidic on mixing (approx. 4.8) as zinc phosphate. There appears to be little irritation to the pulp[18] possibly because there is little penetration of the large polyacrylic acid molecules into the dentine tubules. The liquid for the cement is either a viscous solution of polyacrylic acid or water. If water is used the acid is contained in its anhydrous state within the zinc oxide powder. More recently developed polycarboxylate cements contain fluoride salts, which may aid caries prevention.

Correctly mixed polycarboxylate cement has a consistency similar to that of honey and the cement may appear too viscous to allow proper seating. However, this is normal and should not be of concern since the cement undergoes 'sheer thinning' which reduces the apparent viscosity during the seating of the crown.[19]

Glass ionomer cements
Advantages
- As for polycarboxylate cement but cement has similar acidity to zinc phosphate on mixing
- Fluoride release
Disadvantages
- Sensitive to early moisture contamination
- Low tensile strength
- Not resistant to acid dissolution
- Has been accused of causing post-operative sensitivity but a controlled trial reports it is no worse than zinc phosphate
Recommendations
- Used empirically for conventional crowns where patient has had a previously high caries rate
- May be used as an alternative 'default cement' to zinc phosphate

Conventional glass ionomer cements were first introduced into dentistry as a filling material in 1972.[20] Like polycarboxylates, glass ionomers may be supplied as a powder and aqueous acid (polyalkenoic) or powder and water. The aluminosilicate glass powder of GIC luting cements has smaller particles than GIC filling materials to reduce film thickness, which may be similar to or lower than that of zinc phosphate cements.

For luting purposes, mixing is generally carried out by hand and where provided the manufacturer's powder and liquid dispensers should be used. Encapsulated glass ionomer luting cements are also available and have the advantage of providing the correct powder-liquid ratio.

GIC compares favourably with zinc phosphate with regard to compressive and tensile strength (Table 2). GIC has a significant advantage to zinc phosphate in that it forms a considerable bond to tooth tissue by reaction with the calcium salts in the tooth structure and releases fluoride ions.

The higher solubility in water of GIC in comparison with zinc phosphate and zinc polycarboxylate cements has been identified as a problem when the cement is used for luting purposes. This solubility is adversely affected by early moisture contamination and the cement lute margins should be protected with a varnish following cementation, although this may be difficult when the crown margin is subgingival. Solubility is not a great problem clinically once the cement is set. Another disadvantage of GIC is that its pH during setting is even lower than that of zinc phosphate and some concern has been expressed regarding post-cementation hypersensitivity.[21] However, a randomised, double blind trial of GIC versus zinc phosphate showed no significant difference in sensitivity,[22] but it should be noted that cementation procedures were carefully controlled, including the use of encapsulated mixing. Dentine desiccation may on occasion be responsible for sensitivity; some authorities are convinced that dentinal fluid is drawn into the setting cement, which may cause problems if the preparation is over-dried with an air syringe.

Resin modified glass ionomer cements and compomers
Advantages
- Good compressive and tensile strengths (if correctly proportioned)
- Reasonable working time
- Resistant to water dissolution
- Fluoride release

Disadvantages
- Short track record
- May expand and crack overlying porcelain because of water absorption

Recommendations
- Worth trying for metal or metal ceramic crowns especially where preparation retention is borderline
- Currently unclear which RMGI cements can be used safely with ceramic crowns

Resin modified glass ionomer (RMGI) cements are a hybrid of traditional glass ionomer cement with small additions of light curing resin[23] and generally have the advantages of both in that they are purported to combine the strength and insolubility of resin with the fluoride release of GIC. They were introduced with the aim of overcoming the moisture sensitivity and the low strength of conventional glass ionomers. Examples include Vitremer and Fuji Plus. Compomers are also composed of resin and glass ionomer but are more closely related to composites with the glass ionomer setting reaction occuring slowly as moisture is absorbed into the set resin matrix. Examples include Dyract Cem and Dyract Cem Plus.

The use of RMGIs for luting purposes is becoming more popular because of their relatively high bond strength to dentine, and their ability to form a very thin film layer. RMGIs leach fluoride, but it is unclear how useful this is in preventing secondary caries formation. Several RMGIs are available but whilst they may seem promising clinical studies are still in their infancy. There have also been anecdotal reports of high strength porcelain crowns fracturing following cementation with RMGIs, possibly as a result of expansion of the cement from water sorption.[24] These have been supported by an in-vitro study showing that ceramic crowns crack between 3 and 12 months after cementation with both RMGIs and compomers.[25] RMGIs contain the resin HEMA and absorb significantly more water than composites. In view of these concerns it is best to restrict the use of RMGIs and compomers to metal restorations. Furthermore, when cementing porcelain or composite restorations a better aesthetic result can be achieved with composite resin cements.

Resin cements
Advantages
- Good compressive and tensile strengths
- High tensile strength (relative to conventional cements)
- Resistant to water dissolution
- Relatively resistant to acid dissolution
- Can enhance strength of ceramic restoration if bond obtained

Disadvantages
- Film thickness varies substantially between materials
- Excess material extruded at margin may be difficult to remove especially proximally

Recommendations
- Must be used with or incorporate an effective dentine bonding agent
- Material of choice for porcelain veneers, ceramic onlays and resin bonded ceramic crowns
- May be used to improve retention where preparation geometry sub-optimal, but clinical studies needed to determine long-term success

GLASS IONOMER CEMENTS
A randomised, double blind trial of GIC versus zinc phosphate showed no significant difference in sensitivity

RESIN MODIFIED GLASS IONOMER CEMENTS
Reports of high strength porcelain crowns fracturing following cementation with RMGIs, possibly as a result of expansion of the cement

Resin cements are composites composed of a resin matrix, eg bis-GMA or urethane dimethacrylate, and a filler of fine inorganic particles. They have been available as direct filling materials since the early 1950s[26] but it was not until the early 1970s that a composite resin was introduced for crown and bridge cementation.[27] Resin luting cements differ from restorative composites primarily in their lower filler content and lower viscosity. Following on from their successful use in the cementation of resin bonded bridges and veneers, their popularity has been increasing in recent years for crown cementation because of their use in conjunction with dentine bonding agents (DBA). However even when DBAs are used, resin cements are not without problems (see later).

Composite resin cements are available as self cured, light cured and dual cured materials. The self cured materials are typically used as luting cements because of the inability, or at best difficulty, of light to pass through porcelain and metal restorations. Examples include Panavia,[21] All Bond 2 luting cement and Superbond.

Mechanical and physical properties of resin cements compare favourably with the other cements discussed above (Table 2). In particular, tensile strength is about ten times that of zinc phosphate, which in combination with the high bond strength explains why preparation geometry is of less importance to retention than with conventional cements. This makes resin cements useful for bonding restorations on tooth preparations that would not be retentive enough to succeed with conventional cements. Moreover, a well-bonded composite lute will confer much greater strength to an overlying porcelain restoration than a weaker conventional cement. This feature has been demonstrated *in vitro* with porcelain veneers[28] and *in vivo* with porcelain inlays[29] which were almost five times more likely to fracture when cemented with conventional glass ionomer. It should be noted that effective resin bonding to some high strength porcelain cores (eg In-Ceram) could not be achieved by the usual etching with hydrofluoric acid because of the lack of pores in the material.[30]

Problems with the use of resin cements for luting full crowns include excessive film thickness with some materials,[31,32] marginal leakage because of setting shrinkage, and severe pulpal reactions when applied to cut vital dentine. However, this latter problem may be related more to bacterial infiltration than to any chemical toxicity. The use of DBA under resin cement is critical to its success unless the preparation has been cut only into enamel. Pulpal response is reduced by the use of DBAs, presumably by sealing dentine tubules and reducing microleakage.[33] Adhesive resin cement was found to produce a better marginal seal than zinc phosphate cement.[34] However, even if the problems of microleakage and film thickness could be solved, the problem of adequately removing hardened excess resin from inaccessible margins may preclude the use of resin cement for crowns

with subgingival margins. Indeed, proximal extrusions of resin cement are often radiolucent and may remain undetected.[35]

CROWN CEMENTATION

When a crown has been successfully tried-in and the cement chosen, cementation may then take place. This section will consider conventional cementation. Cementation with resin cements is covered more fully in Parts 12 and 13 of this series on porcelain veneers and resin bonded metal restorations respectively.

Trial cementation

Most dentists are in the habit of fitting crowns and then cementing them with hard cement. Whilst this approach is usually satisfactory there are times where it is difficult to predict a patient's response to changes in aesthetics or occlusion. If such a patient returns unhappy the offending crowns must be cut off – a distressing experience for all concerned. In cases of doubt it is useful to have a period of trial cementation using soft cement, but you must ensure that the definitive restoration can be removed without damage to it or the underlying preparation. To make removal easier the cement should be applied in a ring around the inner aspect of the crown margin. It is important that the manufacturer's modifier is added to the cement. Equal lengths of base and catalyst with a third of a length of modifier will soften cements such as Temp Bond. Alternatively, a 'non-setting' zinc oxide eugenol material (eg Optow Trial Cement) can be used for short periods of soft cementation where preparations are retentive. This material has the advantage that it is easily pealed out of the crown like a membrane, but it cannot be relied upon for more than a few days retention.

Restorations can be removed either by finger pressure or by the application of a matrix band. In cases of difficult removal a Richwil crown remover can be helpful. This crown remover is simply a material, not unlike a sticky sweet, which is softened in hot water, positioned over the crown and the patient asked to bite. Once the material has hardened the crown is removed by asking the patient to snap open. Another way of applying a dislodging force to a soft-cemented crown is to use an impact mallet. The problem with this technique is finding a point of application on the crown. One solution to this problem is to incorporate small lugs resembling mushrooms on the lingual aspect of the crown's metal work.[36] The lugs are removed, of course, prior to hard cementation.

Controlling cement film thickness

The interposition of a cement lute inevitably affects crown seating. Consequently, the art of cementation is to choose a cement with an inherently low film thickness and use techniques which allow it to escape whilst the crown is being seated.

Cement flow can be hindered by preparation features, which cause a build up of hydrostatic

---

RESIN CEMENTS
The tensile strength of resin cements is about ten times that of zinc phosphate

RESIN CEMENTS
The Richwil crown remover is not unlike a sticky sweet

pressure.[37] Thus, retentive preparations, which are long, near parallel and have a large surface area, are most at risk of not seating fully. This problem can be overcome by die spacing and controlled cement application or by venting the crown. These techniques need to be used for all crowns not just apparently retentive ones.

Die spacing is the most common method of achieving space for the cement lute.[38] It involves painting several layers of die relief agent over the whole of the die but avoiding the finish line. The increased cement space results in more rapid seating with decreased deformation of the restoration.[39-41] Die spacing results in a slightly loose fit of a crown on its preparation, but its effect on retention is unclear with some studies reporting an increase in retention[37] while others report a decrease or no effect. A recent study concluded that decreasing the width of the cement layer increases the resistance to dynamic lateral loading.[7] This variability may occur because of differences in cement film thickness. A very thin cement lute may have higher stress concentrations than a slightly thicker one.[42] However, too thick a cement lute is also undesirable as it is liable to fracture.

Another factor which influences the vertical seating of crowns and hence marginal adaptation is the amount of cement loaded into the crown prior to cementation. A study on the effect of volume of zinc phosphate cement, reported that lesser amounts of cement placed within a crown resulted in smaller marginal discrepancy and better occlusal accuracy.[43] Indeed, a crown treated in such a way seated almost 70% better than an identical crown completely filled with cement. However, care must be taken in applying cement in this way not to exceed the working time or the cement may be too viscous at the time of seating.

Venting is an effective[8] but less popular method of reducing cement film thickness. External venting involves creating a perforation in the occlusal surface of the crown, which is sealed with a separate restoration after cementation. With internal venting an escape channel is created either in the axial wall of the preparation or the fit surface of the crown to help cement escape.

The amount of force required to allow maximum seating of cast crowns has been shown to be cement specific.[44] Seating forces are discussed next in relation to cementation technique.

Technique

Isolate the preparation and ensure good moisture control. If the gingivae have overgrown the finish line use either retraction cord with haemostatic agent or if more severe use electrosurgery. A breakdown in technique at any of the following stages will predispose to failure:

- Clean the preparation and crown with water spray
- Air dry but do not desiccate preparation
- Mix cement according to manufacturer's instructions

- Coat the fit surface with cement - do not over-fill
- Only apply cement to preparation if cementing a post

The crown should be seated quickly with firm finger pressure until all excess cement has been expressed from the margins. Seating force must be adequate to ensure complete seating of the crown onto the preparation, but sudden excessive force may result in elastic strain of the dentine, creating a rebound effect, which results in the crown being partly dislodged when the force is removed.[34] Karpidis and Pearson (1988)[45] revealed that crowns seated on preparations in bovine dentine with a force of 300 N/cm² could be removed more easily than those cemented with half the force.

Depending on the angulation of the tooth, pressure may then continue to be exerted onto the crown by the dentist or by the patient biting onto a cotton roll. Some operators prefer a wooden orange stick or similar implement for cementing posterior restorations as this can reduce film thickness. However care must be taken as these are rigid and may only contact part of the occlusal surface of the crown resulting in tipping. Pressure should be maintained for about one minute. Maintaining pressure beyond this time has no appreciable additional effect.[46] It is worth checking the accuracy of the fit at this stage using a sharp probe on the margin and if necessary fine gold margins can be burnished before the cement sets.

Adequate moisture control should be maintained until the cement has set to prevent moisture contamination of the unset material at the crown margin. In the case of conventional cements, excess cement should be left until after the cement sets. For resin-based cements, removal of excess before setting is recommended as it can be very difficult to remove following setting but may still remain despite our best efforts.[47] Some operators apply a smear of petroleum jelly to the outside of the crown which also helps with removal of set cement, but if you do this take great care to prevent contamination of the fit surface. A common failing is for excess cement to be left, especially interproximally. Your nurse can help by having a piece of floss ready. This can be made more effective by tying a knot in the middle of the floss and passing it through the interdental space. Following clean up, a final evaluation of the cemented crown can be made including rechecking the occlusion.

1. Kaufman E G. The retention of crowns before and after cementation. NY Univ J Dent 1967; **25:** 6-7.
2. McClean J W, von Fraunhoffer J A. The estimation of cement film thickness by an in vivo technique. Br Dent J 1971; **131:** 107-111.
3. Christensen G J. Marginal fit of gold inlay castings. J Prosthet Dent 1966; **16:** 297-305.
4. Lang N P, Kiel R A, Anderhalden K. Clinical and microbiological effects of subgingival restorations with overhanging or clinically perfect margins. J Clin Perio 1983; **10:** 563-578.
5. Kelleher M G D, Setchell D J. An investigation of marking materials used in occlusal adjustment. Br Dent J 1984; **156:** 96-102.

6. Monasky G E, Taylor D F. Studies on the wear of porcelain, enamel and gold. *J Prosthet Dent* 1971; **25:** 299-306.
7. Wiskott H W, Belser U C, Scherrer S S. The effect of film thickness and surface texture on the resistance of cemented extracoronal restorations to lateral fatigue. *Int J Prosthodont* 1999; **12:** 255-262.
8. Kaufman E G, Colin L C, Schlagel E, Coelho D H. Factors influencing the retention of cemented gold castings: the cementing medium. *J Prosthet Dent* 1966; **16:** 731-739.
9. Langeland K, Langeland L K. Pulp reactions to crown preparation, impression, temporary crown fixation and permanent cementation. *J Prosthet Dent* 1965; **15:** 129-143.
10. Brännström M, Nyborg H. Bacterial growth and pulpal changes under inlays cemented with zinc phosphate cement and Epoxylite CBA 9080. *J Prosthet Dent* 1974; **31:** 556-565.
11. Brännström M, Nyborg H. Pulpal reaction to polycarboxylate and zinc phosphate cement used with inlays in deep cavity preparations. *J Am Dent Assoc* 1977; **94:** 308-310.
12. Smith D C, Ruse N D. Acidity of glass ionomer cements during setting and its relation to pulp sensitivity. *J Am Dent Assoc* 1986; **112:** 654-657.
13. Chan K C, Svare C W, Horton D J. The effect of varnish on dentinal bonding strength of five dental cements. *J Prosthet Dent* 1976; **35:** 403-406.
14. Brauer G M, McLaughlin R, Huget E F. Aluminium oxide as a reinforcing agent for zinc oxide-eugenol-o-ethoxy-benzoic acid cements. *J Rest Dent* 1968; **47:** 622-628.
15. Phillips R W, Swartz M L, Norman R D, Schnell R J, Niblack B F. Zinc oxide and eugenol cements for permanent cementation. *J Prosthet Dent* 1968; **19:** 144-150.
16. Osbourne J W, Swartz M L, Goodacre C J, Phillips R W, Gale E N. A method for assessing the clinical solubility and disintegration of luting cements. *J Prosthet Dent* 1978; **40:** 413-417.
17. Mesu F P, Reedijk T. Degradation of luting cements measured in vitro and in vivo. *J Rest Dent* 1983; **62:** 1236-1240.
18. Going R E, Mitchem J C. Cements for permanent luting: a summarising review. *J Am Dent Assoc* 1975; **91:** 129-137.
19. Lorton L, Moore M L, Swartz M L, Phillips R W. Rheology of luting cements. *J Rest Dent* 1980; **59:** 1486-1492.
20. Wilson A D, Kent B E. A new translucent cement for dentistry. *Br Dent J* 1972; **132:** 133-135.
21. Smith D C, Ruse N C. Acidity of glass ionomer cements during setting and its relation to pulp sensitivity. *J Am Dent Assoc* 1986; **112:** 654-657.
22. Kern M, Kleimeier B, Schaller H G, Strub J R. Clinical comparison of postoperative sensitivity for a glass ionomer and a zinc phosphate luting cement. *J Prosthet Dent* 1996; **75:** 159-62.
23. Sidhu S K, Watson T F. Resin-modified glass ionomer materials. A status report for the American Journal of Dentistry. *Am J Dent* 1995; **8:** 59-67.
24. Kanchanavista W, Arnstice H M, Pearson G J. Water sorption characteristics of resin-modified glass-ionomer cements. *Biomater* 1997; **18:** 343-349.
25. Leevailoj C, Platt J A, Cochran M A, Moore B K. *In vitro* study of fracture incidence and compressive fracture load of all-ceramic crowns cemented with resin-modified glass ionomer and other luting agents. *J Prosthet Dent* 1998; **80:** 699-707.
26. Schouboe P J, Paffenbarger G C, Sweeney W J. Resin cements and posterior type direct filling resins. *J Am Dent Assoc* 1956; **52:** 584.
27. Lee H, Swartz M L. Evaluation of a composite resin crown and bridge luting agent. *J Rest Dent* 1976; **51:** 756.
28. Brandson S J, King P A. The compact fracture resistance of restored endodontically treated anterior teeth. *J Rest Dent* 1992; **72:** 1141.
29. Åberg C H, van Dijken J W V, Olofsson A-L. Three-year comparison of fired ceramic inlays cemented with composite resin or glass-ionomer cement. *Acta Odontol Scand* 1994; **52:** 140-149.
30. Awliya W, Oden A, Yaman P, Dennison J B, Razzoog M E. Shear bond strength of a resin cement to densely sintered high-purity alumina with various surface conditions. *Acta Odontol Scand* 1998; **56:** 9-13.
31. White S N, Yu Z, Kipnis V. Effect of seating force on film thickness of new adhesive luting agents. *J Prosthet Dent* 1992; **68:** 476-481.
32. White S N, Kipnis V. Effect of adhesive luting agents on the marginal seating of cast restorations. *J Prosthet Dent* 1993; **69:** 28-31.
33. Qvist V, Stolze K, Qvist J. Human pulp reactions to resin restorations performed with different acid-etch restorative procedures. *Acta Odontologica Scandinavia* 1989; **47:** 253-263.
34. Tjan A H L, Dunn J R, Brant B E. Marginal leakage of cast gold crowns luted with an adhesive resin cement. *J Prosthet Dent* 1992; **67:** 11-15.
35. O'Rourke B, Walls A W, Wassell R W. Radiographic detection of overhangs formed by resin composite luting agents. *J Dent* 1995; **23:** 353-357.
36. Pameijer J H N. *Periodontal and occlusal factors in crown and bridge procedures.* pp394. Amsterdam: Centre for Post graduate Courses, 1985.
37. Carter S M, Wilson P R. The effect of die-spacing on crown retention. *Int J Prosthodont* 1996; **9:** 21-29.
38. Grajower R, Zuberi Y, Lewinstein I. Improving the fit of crowns with die spacers. *J Prosthet Dent* 1989; **61:** 555-563.
39. Wilson P R, Goodkind R J, Sakaguchi R. Deformation of crowns during cementation. *J Prosthet Dent* 1990; **64:** 601-609.
40. Wilson P R. The effect of die spacing on crown deformation and seating time. *Int J Prosthodont* 1993; **6:** 397-401.
41. Wilson P R. Effect of increasing cement space on cementation of artificial crowns. *J Prosthet Dent* 1994; **71:** 560-564.
42. Kamposiora P, Papavasilious G, Bayne S C, Felton D A. Finite element analysis estimates of cement microfracture under complete veneer crowns. *J Prosthet Dent* 1994; **71:** 435-441.
43. Tan K, Ibbetson R. The effect of cement volume on crown seating. *Int J Prosthodont* 1996; **9:** 445-451.
44. Wilson P R. Low force cementation. *J Dent* 1996; **24:** 269-273.
45. Karipidis A, Pearson G J. The effect of seating pressure and powder/liquid ratio of zinc phosphate cement on the retention of crowns. *J Oral Rehabil* 1988; **15:** 333-337.
46. Jorgensen K D. Structure of the film thickness of zinc phosphate cements. Factors affecting the film thickness of zinc phosphate. *Acta Odontol Scand* 1960; **18:** 479-501.
47. Mitchell C A, Pintado M R, Geary L, Douglas W H. Retention of adhesive cement on the tooth surface after crown cementation. *J Prosthet Dent* 1999; **81:** 668-677.

List of materials mentioned in text

All Bond 2 dentine bonding agent and luting cement: Bisco Inc, Itasca, IL60143, USA

Dyract Cem and Dyract Cem Plus: Dentsply UK Ltd, Hamm Moor Lane, Addlestone, Weybridge, Surrey KT15 2SE

Fuji Plus: GC, Tokyo, Japan

Premier composite finishing diamonds (white and yellow stripe): Panadent Ltd, 15 Great Dover Street, London SE1 4YW

Kenda polishing points (blue, brown and green for metal; white for porcelain and composite): Austenal Ltd, 4 Crystal Way, Harrow, Middlesex HA1 2HG

Optow Trial Cement: Teledyne Getz, Elkbrook Village, Illinois, USA

Panavia 21: Cavex Holland BV, Haarlem, Holland; supplied by J&S Davis, Summit House, Summit Road, Potters Bar, Hertfordshire EN6 3EE

Richwil Crown and Bridge Remover: Horizon Dental, PO Box 14, Disley, Stockport SK12 2RP

Soflex discs: 3M Health Care Ltd, 3M House, Morley Street, Loughborough

Super Bond: Sun Medical Co Ltd, Moriyama, Japan

Super Diglaze, sub-micron diamond polishing paste: Distributed in UK and Eire by Panadent Ltd, 15 Great Dover Street, London SE1 4YW

Temp Bond: Kerr UK Ltd, Peterborough, UK

Vitremer luting cement: 3M Dental Products, St Paul, Mn, USA

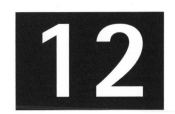

IN BRIEF

- The development of porcelain veneers
- Longevity and factors affecting it
- Tooth preparation, and management of existing restorations
- Impression recording and temporisation (in those few cases which require it)
- Try in, bonding and finishing
- Non-standard porcelain veneers

Crowns and other extra-coronal restorations: Porcelain laminate veneers

A. W. G. Walls[1] J. G. Steele[2] and R. W. Wassell[3]

Porcelain veneers are resin-bonded to the underlying tooth and provide a conservative method of improving appearance or modifying contour, without resorting to a full coverage crown. The porcelain laminate veneer is now a frequently prescribed restoration for anterior teeth. The sums spent by the Dental Practice Board on this type of treatment increased from quarter of a million pounds in 1988/89 to over seven million in 1994/95,[1] representing some 113,582 treatments. Since that time the number has stabilised at over 100,000 veneers prescribed each year.[2] The objective of this paper is to give a practical guide on providing these restorations.

[1*]Professor of Restorative Dentistry,
[2,3]Senior Lecturer in Restorative Dentistry, Department of Restorative Dentistry, The Dental School, Newcastle upon Tyne NE2 4BW;
*Correspondence to: Prof A. W. Walls, Department of Restorative Dentistry, The Dental School, University of Newcastle upon Tyne, Newcastle upon Tyne NE2 4BW
E-mail: a.w.g.walls@ncl.ac.uk

Whenever possible guidelines for provision of porcelain laminate veneers are based on data from the dental literature, but where this is not possible they will be based on our clinical experience and practice. Veneers are often placed on the buccal aspect of maxillary anterior teeth but other applications are possible and these are described at the end of the article.

HISTORY

The concept of veneering was first described in the dental literature some time ago,[3] although it is only with the advent of efficient bonding of resins to enamel and dentine and the use of etched, coupled porcelain surfaces that aesthetically pleasing, durable and successful restorations can be made.[4] These restorations are now an accepted part of the dentist's armamentarium.[5-7] Custom-made acrylic resin veneers preceded them, but these showed unacceptable levels of failure and of marginal stain.[8] Alternative veneering materials are still available, usually either direct or indirect composite resin materials. However, these may suffer from degradation of surface features and accretion of surface stain with time.[9-11]

Porcelain veneers have traditionally been made from aluminous or reinforced feldspathic porcelains, which have relatively poor strength in themselves but produce a strong structure when bonded to enamel. Porcelain veneers can be made from most of the high strength ceramics discussed in the second article of the series. Such materials may hold promise for the future. A study of 83 IPS Empress veneers placed over a 6-year period in private practice reported only one failure, but as yet there are no clinical data

making a direct comparison between these and the traditional materials.

That the strength of traditional porcelain is generally adequate for anterior porcelain veneers is supported by a number of clinical studies. Some authors[9,12-17] have reported low rates of failure because of the loss of retention and fracture (0–5%) with short and medium-term studies of up to 5 years. Indeed, a long-term follow-up[18] of veneers placed over a 10-year period shows a survival rate of 91% at 10.5 years (calculated with the Kaplan Meyer method). These excellent results may, amongst other things, reflect careful case selection, but it is worth noting that other authors,[5,13,19,20] have reported much higher rates of failure of between 7–14% over 2–5 years. Such studies suggest that the risk factors for veneer failure are:

- Bonding onto pre-existing composite restorations (which is considered later)
- Placement by an inexperienced operator
- Using veneers to restore worn or fractured teeth where a combination of parafunction, large areas of exposed dentine and insufficient tooth tissue exist.

Another risk factor, shown up by *in-vitro* work, is the tendency for thermal changes in combination with polymerisation contraction stresses to cause cracking of the veneer when the porcelain is thin and the luting composite thick.[21] A thick composite lute may occur as a result of a poorly fitting veneer or the use of copious die spacer in an attempt to mask underlying tooth discolouration. Least cracking was seen with a ceramic and luting composite thickness ratio above 3.

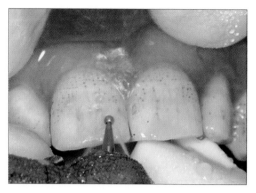

Fig. 1 A 1 mm round diamond bur being used to create depth marks on the buccal surface of UR1 (11)

In-vivo, minor chipping and cracking may be smoothed or repaired without the need to remove the whole veneer. Dunne and Millar reported that the incidence of such repairable defects (8%) was similar to the number of veneers requiring total replacement (11%).[5]

It is useful to be aware of the above data when patients ask how long their proposed veneers are likely to last. It may also be prudent to warn them that although most (80–100%)[7] patients remain satisfied with the aesthetics, veneers are prone to marginal staining, the amount of which will vary from patient to patient. Staining may be caused by one or more of the following:

- Microleakage at the cervical margin, especially where located in aprismatic enamel or, worse still, dentine
- Wear and submargination of the luting composite, especially with an open margin
- Marginal excess of luting composite

To some extent, these factors can be controlled or influenced by careful attention to clinical technique.

CLINICAL TECHNIQUE

A key element in success with porcelain veneers is carefully controlled but appropriate tooth tissue reduction.[22–24] The aims of tooth preparation are to:

- Provide some space into which the technician can build porcelain without over-contouring the tooth
- Provide a finished preparation that is smooth and has no sharp internal line-angles which would give areas of high stress concentration in the restoration
- Maintain the preparation within enamel whenever possible
- Define a finish line to which the technician can work.

It may be possible to prepare veneer preparations without local anaesthetic. However, in our experience, sub-gingival margin placement, inadvertent dentine exposure and the unpleasant coldness from the water spray and aspirator usually make its use advisable.

Depth of preparation

It is desirable for the tooth preparation to remain within enamel so careful control of preparation depth is important. Obviously, the enamel thickness varies from the incisal edge to the cervical margin. Hence the preparation depth will need to vary over the length of the tooth to avoid (if possible) exposing dentine. The preparation depth should be of the order of 0.4 mm close to the gingival margin, rising to 0.7 mm for the bulk of the preparation. This is best achieved by using a depth mark of some sort. In our experience formal depth grooves can be of limited value in this area as there is a tendency for the bur to catch and run into the groove during buccal reduction, accentuating the groove. The alternative is to use depth pits prepared on the surface of the tooth using a 1 mm diameter round bur sunk to half its diameter (Fig. 1). The buccal surface reduction can then be undertaken to join the base of the pits. The reduction should mimic the natural curvature of the tooth in order to provide an even thickness of porcelain layer over the tooth surface, hence it should be in at least two planes.[24]

When the tooth concerned is markedly discoloured, it is sensible to undertake a greater level of reduction to give the technician more chance to mask the underlying stain without over-contouring the tooth. This will have obvious disadvantages, as the preparation is likely to extend into dentine with greater depth of tooth reduction.

Nattrass *et al.*[25] have demonstrated that even with experienced operators and careful control of cutting instruments there is a tendency for dentine to be exposed in the cervical and proximal regions of the preparations, where the enamel is thinnest. This should be borne in mind when deciding on the type of luting agent to be used in veneer placement. They also found that there was a tendency for variations in tooth preparation depth across their samples with least reduction in the mid-incisal region. There is no suggestion in the literature as yet that this causes any long-term damage to the tooth or affects the longevity of the veneer.

Incisal edge reduction

One important decision to make before commencing the preparation is whether or not the incisal edge of the tooth is to be reduced. There are four basic preparation designs that have been described for the incisal edge (Fig. 2):

- *Window,* in which the veneer is taken close to but not up to the incisal edge. This has the advantage of retaining natural enamel over the incisal edge, but has the disadvantage that the incisal edge enamel is weakened by the preparation. Also, the margins of the veneer would become vulnerable if there is incisal edge wear whilst the incisal lute can be difficult to hide.
- *Feather,* in which the veneer is taken up to the height of the incisal edge of the tooth but the edge is not reduced. This has the advantage that once again guidance on natural tooth is maintained but the veneer is liable to be fragile at the incisal edge and may be subject to peel/sheer forces during protrusive guidance.
- *Bevel,* in which a bucco-palatal bevel is prepared across the full width of the preparation

and there is some reduction of the incisal length of the tooth. This gives more control over the incisal aesthetics and a positive seat during try in and luting of the veneer. The margin is not in a position that will be subjected to direct shear forces except in protrusion. However, this style of preparation does involve more extensive reduction of tooth tissue.

- *Incisal overlap,* in which the incisal edge is reduced and then the veneer preparation extended onto the palatal aspect of the preparation. This also helps to provide a positive seat for luting whilst involving more extensive tooth preparation. This style of preparation will also modify the path of insertion of the veneer which will have to be seated from the buccal/incisal direction rather than the buccal alone. Care needs to be taken to ensure that any proximal wrap around of the preparation towards the gingival margin does not produce an undercut to the desired path of insertion for the veneer. It may be necessary to rotate such veneers into place by locating the incisal edge first then rotating the cervical margin into position.

There is little data available upon which to base a decision over incisal edge preparation. Hui *et al.*[26] demonstrated that veneers in window preparations were best able to resist incisal edge loading and that an overlap design fractured at the lowest loads. However, the magnitude of loading at which the overlap design veneers failed was much greater than that encountered clinically for such teeth. Furthermore, a clinical study was unable to distinguish any difference in failure rate between incisal preparation designs after two and a half years of service.[27] If the operator intends to either improve the incisal edge aesthetics or to increase the length of a tooth then either an overlap or bevel design would be the preparation of choice. If it were not necessary to extend the incisal edges, then it may be possible to use a feather-edge design, however the operator has less control of incisal edge aesthetics with this approach. Nordbo *et al.*[14] report no failures but 5% incisal chipping at 3-years for veneers placed using a feather-edge design and 0.3 to 0.5 mm buccal tooth reduction.

The authors would not recommend the buccal window, as it is very difficult to mask the incisal finish line of the restoration. As this style of restoration is used to improve the appearance of teeth, the introduction of an aesthetic defect would be inappropriate. If the incisal edge is to be modified then the length should be reduced by some 0.5–0.75 mm[28] to allow adequate strength within the porcelain incisal edge without elongating the tooth. Depth grooves can be used to monitor accurately incisal edge reduction (Fig. 1); we would strongly recommend this approach.

Axial tooth reduction

Axial tooth reduction is best undertaken using diamond burs in either an airotor or a speed

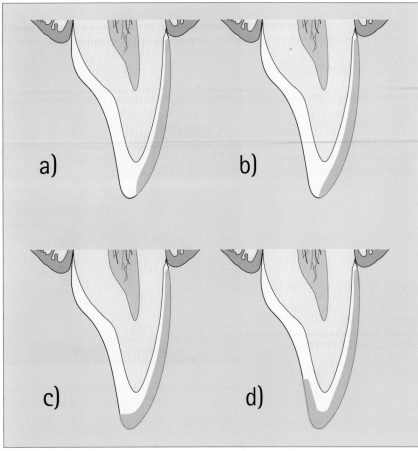

Fig. 2 Four incisal preparations are possible for veneers: a) window , b) feather , c) bevel or d) incisal overlap

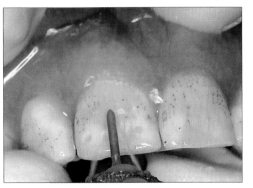

Fig. 3 Straight sided torpedo-shaped diamond bur provides more predictable axial reduction in association with depth marks than a flame-shaped bur

accelerating handpiece with a conventional motor. It is easier to achieve predictable tooth reduction using either a parallel sided or tapered bur with straight sides rather than a flame-shaped bur (Fig. 3). Some clinicians advocate preparing the gingival finish line as the first step using a round diamond bur of appropriate diameter, which will automatically produce a chamfered finish line. Alternatively a torpedo shaped bur can be used to produce both the axial reduction and the gingival finish line (Fig. 4), which is the method we prefer.

Conventional diamond burs leave a macroscopically roughened surface on enamel. Further preparation of the tooth using either a small particle size diamond bur or a multi-fluted tungsten carbide finishing bur will smooth the surface of the preparation and can be used to refine the finishing margin. At this stage the gingival tissues

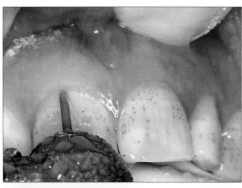

Fig. 4 The torpedo bur can also be used to create the gingival bevel

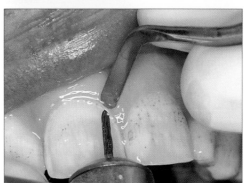

Fig. 5 A flat plastic instrument protects the gingivae during finishing of the chamfer with a multi-fluted tungsten carbide bur. A speed accelerating handpiece provides greater control than an airotor

can be protected from damage using a flat plastic instrument (Fig. 5) or gingival retraction cord can be packed for the same purpose, which will in turn facilitate the impression. It is often impractical to provide provisional restorations for porcelain veneers (see later) but some patients are conscious of the roughened tooth surface in their mouths, which should be smoothed.

Proximal finish lines
It is best if the proximal finishing margins for the preparation do not extend beyond the contact point in the incisal third of the tooth – in other words, the contact point with adjacent teeth should be maintained. If it proves necessary to prepare through the contact area then some form of provisional restoration would be required to prevent inadvertent tooth movement between tooth preparation and fitting of the veneers. Cervically it may be necessary to extend the preparation into the gingival embrasure to mask discoloured tooth substance in the proximal zone immediately above the interdental papilla. Care must be used not to create an undercut preparation in this area to the proposed path of insertion of the restoration.

It is usually necessary to trim the proximal finish line with a chisel to avoid the sharp lip of enamel that often results from being unable to take the bur to the very edge of the preparation. In this respect it is better to change to a smaller diameter bur to prepare the proximal margins of a single tooth being veneered to permit limited tooth reduction without damaging the adjacent tooth.

Cervical finish lines
The cervical finish lines for a veneer should be a chamfer with about a 0.4 mm maximum depth.

The rounded internal line angle will help to reduce stresses in the margin of the veneer that may otherwise develop during firing. Also, porcelain will adapt more readily to this shape during manufacture. The finish line should lie just at the crest of the free gingival margin, unless the veneers are being used to mask severe staining when greater sub-gingival extension may be required for aesthetic reasons. This position for the gingival extension of the veneer usually gives the best compromise between aesthetic control of the finished restoration and the ease with which the clinician can control moisture during luting.

It is helpful to have a defined cervical finishing margin so that the porcelain technician will be able to identify clearly the desired extent of the veneer. However, there is a tendency for the cervical margins of finished veneers to be over-bulked to give greater durability during clinical handling. These margins should therefore be thinned as well as finished after luting.

Coping with pre-existing restorations
Some teeth that require veneers will have existing composite resin restorations in place. There are two ways to deal with this:

- *Bond to a prepared composite resin surface.* This is difficult, particularly if the composite restoration has been in place for any length of time. Water sorption, exposed un-silanated surfaces of filler particles and limited opportunities for further polymerisation of the resin component of the set material all contribute to a reduced bond strength.
- *Replace the restoration.* This can be done relatively easily, but should be done at the visit when the veneer is luted to the tooth so the new composite has the best chance of bonding to the porcelain veneer as well as the tooth tissue. This makes the procedure for bonding the veneer more complex. The old restoration needs to be removed before the veneer is attached to the tooth. The veneer is then luted in place using the requisite bonding system and subsequently the composite resin restoration replaced in the same manner as when placing a conventional Class III or IV composite filling. It can be difficult to avoid producing overhanging margins using this technique, so care is required to ensure that any such overhangs are identified and eliminated.

One of the causes for failure that Dunne and Millar[5] identified was that veneers were attached to pre-existing restorations. It would seem sensible to replace such restorations at the time of veneer placement to reduce this as a possible cause of early failure of the veneer. Alternatively, if there are extensive restorations present it may be more sensible to provide a crown.

Recording an impression
Impression technique and soft tissue handling are dealt with elsewhere in this series, so we will not go into great detail here. However it is

appropriate to use short sections of retraction cord around the margins of the preparations to facilitate the capture of both the finishing edge of the preparation and the adjacent area of unprepared tooth. Electro-surgery is best avoided because of the risk of gingival recession revealing the veneer margin.

An impression of the opposing arch is indispensable if the incisal edges of the veneers are involved in guidance.

Laboratory prescription and manufacture
Again, communication with your technician and achieving maximum aesthetics is covered elsewhere in this series. Of particular importance in relation to veneers is careful shade selection, especially if you are planning to modify the colour of the tooth. If you intend to attempt to modify the shade of the veneer with the luting agent then it is sensible to ask the technician to provide space for the luting resin using a proprietary die-spacing system but bear in mind that the porcelain should not be so thin that there is a risk of it being cracked by the thick composite lute.[21] In addition, if a diagnostic wax-up has been used to demonstrate a modification in anterior aesthetics then this should be sent to the laboratory as well. It can also be beneficial to send a study cast of the teeth prior to preparation if one is available should you want to preserve the original tooth form.

There are a variety of methods for manufacture of porcelain veneers using either a refractory die material, a platinum matrix laid down on a conventional working model or one of the castable ceramic materials prepared using the lost wax technique. Sim and Ibbetson[29] have shown that the best quality of marginal fit was obtained with a platinum foil system, followed by a refractory die and that the worst fit was associated with cast glass restorations.

It is best to ask your laboratory for the veneer to be etched with hydrofluoric acid but not to apply the silane-coupling agent. These agents need to be applied just prior to luting the veneer in place (whether or not the laboratory has applied silane) and are provided in most commercially available resin luting kits. Too early an application of a coupling agent, or contamination of the coupling agent coated surface prior to bonding can reduce the strength of the attachment between resin and veneer. Also, two component silane systems must not be kept after mixing as the silane polymerises to an unreactive polysiloxane, again with a reduction in bond strength.[7]

Provisional restorations
It is difficult and time-consuming to provide provisional restorations for teeth prepared for porcelain veneers. It is often best simply to leave the teeth in their prepared state providing the patient is aware that this is going to happen and the teeth are not sensitive.

A variety of techniques have been described for placement of provisional restorations if they are required. These include directly placed composite resin veneers and producing a transparent matrix from a thermoplastic material to allow multiple composite veneers to be made simultaneously.[30] Such provisional restorations need to be attached to the enamel surface and the only practical way to do this is using the acid etch technique. Obviously, only a very small area of enamel in the centre of the preparation should be spot-etched to provide attachment for the composite resin, which can then be removed easily during the next visit without damaging the periphery of the preparation. It is best to avoid the margins of the preparations when doing this with spot etching at the centre only.

Provisional restorations should be made with care, avoiding gingival excess. Any such excess would cause gingival irritation whilst the veneers are being made and may result in an alteration of the position of the gingival margin or cause difficulty with bleeding during luting.

Provisional restorations are useful when you plan to alter the position of the teeth using veneers. The diagnostic wax-up can be used to prepare a thermoplastic matrix. This matrix is then used to make composite resin veneers directly in the mouth. This will allow the patient to experience the planned changes to their teeth at first hand and to approve the change in their appearance before the definitive restorations are made, avoiding a potential cause for grievance.

Trial placement. The veneers should be returned from the laboratory in a foam-lined box rather than on the working model of the patient. It is important that neither you nor the laboratory place the etched veneers back on the stone dies. Any contact between the etched porcelain surface and dental stone will result in abrasion of the stone model and some stone dust becoming trapped in the delicate veneer surface. Swift *et al.*[31] have shown that such contamination results in a substantial fall in the bond strength between veneer and resin. They also found that it was very difficult to clean an etched porcelain surface that has been contaminated with dental stone.

Handling porcelain veneers can be difficult; they are small and delicate. There are commercially available devices to help with this, either in the form of a tiny suction cup or a small rod with a tacky resin at one end. Alternatively a little piece of ribbon wax on the end of an amalgam plugger makes a useful substitute.

Check the quality of fit and gingival extension of the veneer against the tooth, which should have been cleaned with pumice in water prior to the trial. Once you are happy that the quality of fit is acceptable, the next stage is to assess the colour match. The colour of a porcelain veneer cannot be assessed if the veneer is simply placed on the surface of the tooth. Much of the overall colour for the final restoration comes from the tooth structure, so a colour-coupling agent is needed between the tooth and the veneer (Fig. 6).

In its simplest form water will allow the colour of the tooth to be expressed through the

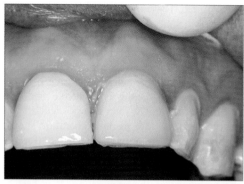

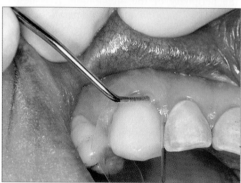

veneer and give a reasonable guide to the overall appearance if a neutral coloured luting resin is to be used.

If it is necessary to try to modify the colour of the finished restoration using the luting resin then the veneer must be tried in with an appropriate colour of paste. This can either be the luting agent itself or, alternatively, some manufacturers provide trial pastes that will not set but have similar optical properties to the luting resin. If the definitive luting resin is used great care must be taken to ensure that the resin does not set under the action of the operating light and that the paste used for the trial is removed completely from the veneer. Some manufacturer's trial pastes are water-soluble making their removal relatively straightforward. However if a resin based trial paste is used this needs to be removed using an organic solvent. Swift et al.[31] found that acetone, an agent that has often been suggested and used for this role, produces markedly reduced bond strengths. A more acceptable alternative would be ethanol. Once the quality of fit of the veneer and the shade of the luting paste have been assessed the etched surface of the porcelain should be coated with a silane coupling agent, following the manufacturer's instructions for the product chosen.

Luting the veneer
Having established that the veneer is of an appropriate shade, or can be modified with a luting resin to be satisfactory, it is ready to be bonded to the supporting enamel and dentine. In view of the reported high prevalence of dentine exposure on veneer preparations[25] we would advise the routine use of a dentine bonding agent.

Good moisture control is critical if adhesive techniques are to work. Contamination of either the prepared tooth surface or the veneer fitting surface with saliva, blood or crevicular fluid will result in reduced bond strengths. Moisture control can be achieved using rubber dam, but where this is impractical gingival retraction cord can be a helpful adjunct to prevention of contamination from the gingival crevice. The residual enamel should be cleaned using pumice and water and then etched, washed and dried. Details of technique will not be given here, as they are so material specific. It can be tempting to cut corners during this stage, but it is vital that you use the luting resins as the manufacturer suggests to achieve optimal results.

Having applied the dentine/enamel bonding system the veneer should be loaded with luting resin and located on the surface of the tooth. At this stage the excess of unset resin around the periphery of the veneer can best be removed using a metal instrument (Fig. 7) or a brush dipped in unfilled resin. Removal needs to be undertaken with care, as there is a tendency for resin to be pulled out from the periphery of the lute space leaving sub-margination, particularly if dental floss is used.

Once all gross excess is removed the luting resin can be cured using a visible light activation unit. It is essential to ensure an adequate exposure to cure fully the luting resin through the porcelain veneer. Most manufacturers' guidelines suggest 30–40s cure times. This is inadequate with research suggesting that 60s is more realistic.[32–34]

Light-activation of a luting agent through an opaque veneer or one of greater than 0.7 mm thickness, is not adequately effective.[35] In these circumstances a dual-curing resin, which is initiated both by admixing the pastes to give a chemical set and by visible-light activation, should be used. Such dual-cure agents should not be used on thinner veneers as they do not polymerise as effectively as a visible-light activated equivalent alone and may be susceptible to colour change with time as a product of the residue of the chemical initiating system.[36]

Post placement finishing
The final stage for any restoration is finishing the margins of the restoration and any functional contacts to give a smooth and harmonious transition from tooth to restoration. It is particularly important to eliminate any occlusal interferences. The finishing process for porcelain veneers involves using small particle size diamond burs or multi-fluted tungsten carbide burs in either an airotor or a speed accelerating handpiece (Fig. 8). Burs are available in a variety of grit sizes to polish the margins progressively and ideally should be followed by the use of 10 mm particle size diamond polishing paste to maximise the lustre on the porcelain and the cement lute (Fig. 9). Finishing can also be achieved using rotating abrasive disks that are available for composite resin restorations (eg Soflex discs, Super-Snaps etc).

When finishing the gingival extent of the veneer it is sensible to protect the gingival tissues using a flat plastic instrument. You will want to show the finished result to your patient, who will not be impressed if the gingival tissues are lacerated and bleeding! Many operators prefer to delay the detailed finishing until a subsequent appointment at which time any excess material is much easier to identify.

NON-STANDARD VENEERS

Veneers are generally prescribed for the buccal aspects of maxillary anterior teeth, but there are a number of 'non-standard' applications. These include veneers for:

- The palatal/lingual aspect of teeth which have been worn or fractured
- Diastema elimination using slips restricted to the proximal aspects of teeth
- Lower incisors
- Posterior occlusal onlays

All of these applications require some careful thought to ensure a satisfactory result.

Palatal veneers

There are two main problems with palatal veneers.

Firstly, it is not possible to adjust the occlusal contacts on the veneer until it is luted in place. This will inevitably result in the need to adjust porcelain in situ. When this is required it is *essential* that the adjusted porcelain surface be polished with graded abrasives, culminating in diamond paste, to ensure that the opposing teeth are not subject to excessive wear from roughened unglazed porcelain.

Secondly, the finish line for such veneers often extends onto the buccal surface of the tooth. It can be very difficult to disguise that line as the resin luting agent can prove highly visible at the junction between porcelain and tooth (Fig. 10). One option is to try to hide the finish line as much as possible. There are three ways to improve this:

- Never make the finish line a straight line. The human eye is very good at identifying straight lines, but is less good at seeing wavy lines. If the finish line is made serpentinous, using the normal anatomy of the tooth to rise over the mamelons and dip between them, it becomes more difficult to see (Fig. 11).
- Extend the finish line over onto the buccal surface of the tooth significantly. Then ask your technician to gradually increase the quantity of translucent porcelain in the overlapping section so that more and more colour from the restoration is drawn from the tooth and less and less from the veneer. This avoids sudden change in optical properties between tooth and porcelain restoration. (Figs 10, 11)
- Use a luting agent that is colour neutral with the tooth so that it blends as much as possible.

Lateral porcelain slips

There are once again two problems with this sort of porcelain addition, commonly used to obliterate a diastema between teeth.

- Care must be taken to avoid a bulky gingival emergence profile. It is not acceptable to pro-

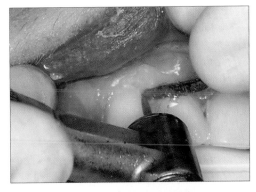

Fig. 8 Finishing the gingival margin of the veneer with a small particle size diamond bur in a speed accelerating handpiece. Once again, a flat plastic instrument protects the gingival tissues

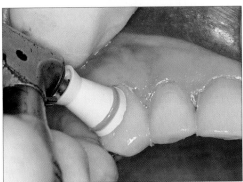

Fig. 9 Final polishing of the gingival margin of the veneer using a rubber cup and diamond polishing paste

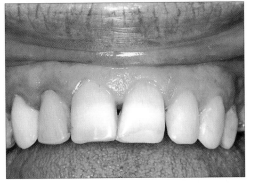

Fig. 10 Unsightly, porcelain-tooth junctions at the incisal overlap of the palatal surface veneers at UL1, UL2 and UL3 (21, 22 and 23). The junctions are clearly visible due to the abrupt change in optical contrast and the straight finish line

duce artificial overhangs that are not cleansable and are liable to act as plaque traps.
- The junction between porcelain and tooth should be disguised. This is best hidden within the natural anatomy of the tooth by placing the finish line within the intermamelon groove closest to the addition and by using the same concepts as above to blend tooth and porcelain. In this circumstance it may be possible to have a straight finish line, at worst it mimics a crack on the crown surface.

An alternative is simply to extend the veneer over the whole buccal surface with an appropriate extension into the proximal space.

Veneers for mandibular incisors

Mandibular incisors can be managed with porcelain veneers but the preparation usually has to be extended over the incisal edge of the tooth, particularly if the tooth is in functional contact. The incisal coverage of porcelain has to be sufficiently thick to be durable under continuing rubbing contact with the opposing tooth. This would necessitate incisal edge reduction by between 0.75 and 1 mm. Obviously if the tooth is not temporised there is a risk of over-eruption of

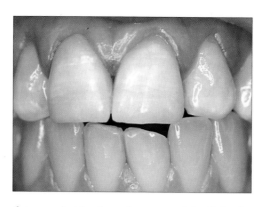

Fig. 11 Here the incisal overlap has been hidden. The palatal veneers on UR1 (11) and UL1 (21) have had their incisal margins extended some 2mm onto the buccal surface of the tooth with a gradual increase in translucency of the porcelain to improve colour transmission. Also, the finish line is serpentinous

the opposing tooth or the prepared tooth in the period between preparation and fit of the veneers. Space maintenance is best provided by adding composite resin to the palatal surface of the upper teeth to produce a stable occlusal stop between the upper and lower arches, rather than risking damage to the prepared enamel surface of the lower.

Posterior occlusal onlays

Porcelain occlusal onlays (sometimes termed 'shims') have the potential to offer an elegant and aesthetic means of reconstructing the occlusal surfaces of worn or broken-down teeth. However, despite the initial enthusiasm of some authors[37] the results with traditional aluminous or feldspathic porcelains have proved disappointing. We have experienced both debonding and fracture, especially when restorations are attached mainly to dentine, and subject to the rigors of bruxism. It may be that one or more of the high strength ceramics would be suitable for this purpose,[38] but it is too early to make any firm recommendations.

CONCLUSIONS

Porcelain veneers are a useful adjunct to the armamentarium of the dentist to help in the management of aesthetic problems in patients, both young and old. Care needs to be taken during tooth preparation and particularly during the luting phase to ensure maximal results are obtained for the patient.

1. DPB. *Dental Data Digest of Statistics*. Dental Practice Board, 1996.
2. DPB. *Dental Data Digests of Statistics for 1997, 1998, 1999, 2000 and 2001*. Dental Practice Board, 2001.
3. Pincus C. Building mouth personality. *Alpha Omega* 1948; **42**: 163-166.
4. Horn H R. Porcelain veneers. Dental Clinics of North America 1983; **27**: 671-684.
5. Dunne S M, Millar B J. A longitudinal study of the clinical performance of porcelain veneers. *Br Dent J* 1993; **175**: 317-321.
6. Guidelines. Restorative indications for porcelain veneer restorations. *In:* Gregg T, editor. *Faculty of Dental Surgery National Clinical Guidelines*. London: Faculty of Dental Surgeons of Royal College of Surgeons of England, 1997.
7. Peumans M, Van Meerbeek B, Lambrechts P, Vanherle G. Porcelain veneers: a review of the literature. *J Dent* 2000; **28**: 163-77.
8. Walls A W G, Murray J J, McCabe J F. Composite laminate veneers: a clinical study. *J Oral Rehabil* 1988; **15**: 439-454.
9. Rucker L M R W, MacEntee M, Richardson A,. Porcelain and resin veneers clinically evaluated: 2-year results. *J Am Dent Assoc* 1990; **121**: 594-596.
10. Harley K E, Ibbetson R J. Anterior veneers for the adolescent patient: 1. General indications and composite veneers. *Dent Update* 1991; **18**: 55-6, 58-9.
11. Welbury R R. A clinical study of a microfilled composite resin for labial veneers. *Int J Paed Dent* 1991; **1**: 9-15.
12. Clyde J, Gilmoure A. Porcelain veneers: a preliminary review. *Br Dent J* 1988; **164**: 9-14.
13. Strassler H, Nathanson D. Clinical evaluation of etched porcelain veneers over a period of 18-42 months. *J Aesthet Dent* 1989; **1**: 21-28.
14. Nordbo H, Rygh-Thoresen N, Henaug T. Clinical performance of porcelain laminate veneers without incisal overlapping: 3-year results. *J Dent* 1994; **22**: 342-345.
15. Peumans M, Van Meerbeek B, Lambrechts P, Vuylsteke-Wauters M, Vanherle G. Five-year clinical performance of porcelain veneers. *Quintessence Int* 1998; **29**: 211-221.
16. Kihn P, Barnes D. The clinical evaluation of porcelain veneers: a 48-month clinical evaluation. *J Am Dent Assoc* 1998; **129**: 747-752.
17. Fradeani M. Six-year follow-up with Empress veneers. *Int J Periodont Rest Dent* 1998; **18**: 216-225.
18. Dumfahrt H, Schaffer H. Porcelain laminate veneers. A retrospective evaluation after 1 to 10 years of service: Part II—Clinical results. *Int J Prosthodont* 2000; **13**: 9-18.
19. Christensen G, Christensen R. Clinical observations of porcelain veneers. *J Aesthet Dent* 1991; **3**: 174-179.
20. Walls A W. The use of adhesively retained all-porcelain veneers during the management of fractured and worn anterior teeth: Part 2. Clinical results after 5 years of follow-up. *Br Dent J* 1995; **178**: 337-40.
21. Magne P, Kwon K R, Belser U C, Hodges J S, Douglas W H. Crack propensity of porcelain laminate veneers: A simulated operatory evaluation. *J Prosthet Dent* 1999; **81**: 327-334.
22. Calamia J R. Materials and techniques for etched porcelain facial veneers. *Alpha Omega* 1988; **81**: 48-51.
23. Garber D. Traditional tooth preparation for porcelain laminate veneers. *Comp Cont Ed Dent* 1991; **12**: 316, 318, 320, 322.
24. Harley K E, Ibbetson R. Anterior veneers for the adolescent patient: 2 Porcelain veneers and conclusions. *Dent Update* 1991; **18**: 112-116.
25. Nattrass B R, Youngson C C, Patterson C J, Martin D M, Ralph J P. An *in vitro* assessment of tooth preparation for porcelain veneer restorations. *J Dent* 1995; **23**: 165-170.
26. Hui K, Williams B, Davis E, Holt R. A comparative assessment of the strengths of porcelain veneers for incisor teeth dependent on their design characteristics. *Br Dent J* 1991; **171**: 51-55.
27. Meijering A C, Creugers N H, Roeters F J, Mulder J. Survival of three types of veneer restorations in a clinical trial: a 2.5-year interim evaluation. *J Dent* 1998; **26**: 563-568.
28. Calamia J. Materials and techniques for etched porcelain facial veneers. *Alpha Omega* 1988; **81**: 48-51.
29. Sim C, Ibbetson R J. Comparison of fit of porcelain veneers fabricated using different techniques. *Int J Prosthodont* 1993; **6**: 36-42.
30. Raigrodski A J, Sadan A, Mendez A J. Use of a customized rigid clear matrix for fabricating provisional veneers. *J Esthet Dent* 1999; **11**: 16-22.
31. Swift B, Walls A W, McCabe J F. Porcelain veneers: the effects of contaminants and cleaning regimens on the bond strength of porcelain to composite. *Br Dent J* 1995; **179**: 203-208.
32. Strang R, McCrossan J, Muirhead M, Richardson S. The setting of visible light cured resins beneath etched porcelain veneers. *Br Dent J* 1987; **163**: 149-151.
33. Warren K. An investigation into the microhardness of a light-cured composite when cured through varying thicknesses of porcelain. *J Oral Rehabil* 1990; **17**: 327-334.
34. O'Keefe K, Pease P, Herren H. Variables affecting the spectral transmittance of porcelain through porcelain veneer samples. *J Prosthet Dent* 1991; **66**: 434-438.
35. Linden J J, Swift E J, Jr., Boyer D B, Davis B K. Photo-activation of resin cements through porcelain veneers. *J Dent Res* 1991; **70**: 154-157.
36. Berrong J M, Weed R M, Schwartz I S. Color stability of selected dual-cure composite resin cements. *J Prosthodont* 1993; **2**: 24-27.
37. Mabrito C, Roberts M. Porcelain onlays. *Curr Opin Cosmetic Dent* 1995: 1-8.
38. Denissen H, Dozic A, van der Zel J, van Waas M. Marginal fit and short-term clinical performance of porcelain-veneered CICERO, CEREC, and Procera onlays. *J Prosthet Dent* 2000; **84**: 506-13.

IN BRIEF

- The indications for the management of worn teeth, in occlusal management, and following molar endodontics
- Design and tooth preparation for anterior and posterior teeth
- Clinical procedures, including management of existing restorations and bonding
- Problems with aesthetics and temporisation
- Maintenance and, where necessary, rebonding

Crowns and other extra-coronal restorations: Resin-bonded metal restorations

A. W. G. Walls[1] F. S. A. Nohl[2] and R. W. Wassell[3]

Resin-bonded metal restorations is the final part of the series. Cast metal restorations which rely on adhesion for attachment to teeth are attractive because of their potential to be much more conservative of tooth structure than conventional crowns which rely on preparation features providing macromechanical resistance and retention.

[1]Professor of Restorative Dentistry, [3]Senior Lecturer in Restorative Dentistry, Department of Restorative Dentistry, The School of Dental Sciences, Framlington Place, Newcastle upon Tyne NE2 4BW [2]Consultant in Restorative Dentistry, The Dental Hospital, Richardson Road, Newcastle upon Tyne NE2 4SZ
*Correspondence to: Prof A. W. G. Walls, Department of Restorative Dentistry, The Dental School, University of Newcastle upon Tyne, Newcastle upon Tyne NE2 4BW
E-mail: a.w.g.walls@ncl.ac.uk

The past 25 years have witnessed great strides in the development of adhesive dentistry. Many would say that our day-to-day practice has been influenced more fundamentally by these advances than by any other recent dental innovation.

One of the advances is the introduction of resin-bonded metal restorations (RBMR). Anteriorly, the RBMR resembles a retentive wing of a resin-bonded minimal preparation bridge. Posteriorly, the RBMR (sometimes termed a shim) resembles a conventional metal onlay but usually without box forms or other mechanical means of providing retention. Sometimes however, where pre-existing restorations have been replaced as part of the RBMR, the distinction between onlay and shim becomes blurred; the only differentiation being the means of cementation which has evolved from the technology developed for resin-bonded bridgework.

The need to remove tooth substance to achieve mechanical resistance and retention of worn teeth for conventional crowns would seem particularly counterproductive: RBMR can offer conservative solutions in this situation. A number of case reports and two surveys[1,2] have appeared documenting and supporting the use of RBMR on the palatal aspects of worn maxillary anterior teeth (Fig. 1). The use of RBMR on the occlusal surfaces of posteriors has also been described (Fig. 2).[2–4] However, there are no well-controlled clinical studies of the long-term success of RBMR in comparison with conventional restorations. Other uses have included production of rests for the support of partial dentures[5] and restorations to alter the morphology of occlusal holding and guiding surfaces of canines.[6]

The ability to bond cast metal alloys to teeth

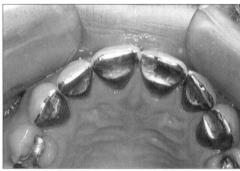

Fig. 1 Occlusal view of anterior palatal resin-bonded metal restorations

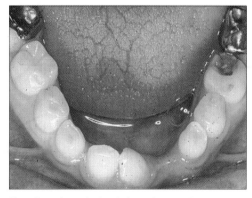

Fig. 2 Posterior resin-bonded metal restoration

was first demonstrated clinically by Rochette in 1973.[7] His periodontal splint was made of cast gold and retained macromechanically by composite resin extruded through countersunk perforations in the metalwork. Tooth surfaces were etched with acid to provide micromechanical retention for composite resin cement. The major breakthrough was that other than etching no destructive tooth preparation was required.

As the adhesive minimal preparation bridge became commonplace, methods of modifying base metal alloys were developed to improve adhesion of the retainers to tooth substance via a resin-based cement. One technique was to incorporate irregularities into the fitting surface of the retainers during pattern formation, which were subsequently reproduced in metal; these took the form of voids left after the wash out of salt crystals, spheres or meshwork, but had the disadvantage that castings were bulky and the laboratory technique was exacting. Microscopic etch patterns in the fitting surface of bridge retainers greatly increase the surface area for contact with luting agents and can be produced by electrolytic corrosion in an acidic environment. Again this approach was technique sensitive but could produce reliable attachment between metals and resin.[8] Base metal retainers can also be air abraded with alumina particles that as well as increasing the surface area may enhance the bond with some cements by chemical interactions.[9]

Lesser demands on rigidity with single unit restorations enabled the use of precious metal alloys (type III gold [ADA classification]) rather than the nickel based alloys used in adhesive bridgework. This gives advantages in casting accuracy, ease of adjustment and finishing, the potential for reduced wear of opposing teeth and perhaps of appearance. Several precious metal surface treatments have been documented. These include tin plating,[9] heat treatment of high copper content gold alloys,[10] air abrasion of the cast metal surface,[2,10] and the Silicoater.[11] Air abraded base metal luted to etched enamel using two chemically active cements gave higher bond strengths *in-vitro* than precious metal alloy/surface treatment combinations.[9] However, tin plating or heat treating air abraded precious metal alloys gave enhanced bond strengths *in-vitro* compared with this alloy air abraded alone.[10] Clinically, air abraded nickel-chromium anterior RBMRs cemented with Panavia Ex gave a survival probability of 0.74 at 56 months,[1] and air-abraded gold RBMRs (anterior and posterior), also cemented with Panavia Ex, were associated with a survival probability of 89% at 60 months.[2] However it cannot be assumed that because a metal surface treatment works with one cement that it will necessarily be effective with others.

INDICATIONS

In the management of worn teeth
RBMR can protect worn and vulnerable tooth surfaces from the effects of further wear by forming a barrier against mechanical and chemical insults.

Any technique, which could delay entry into a restorative spiral necessitating ever enlarging restorations with endodontic implications, is to be welcomed. Although RBMR are susceptible to debonding, marginal recurrent caries and marginal lute wear, the fact that little if any tooth preparation has been carried out prior to placement means that cumulative insults to the pulp are likely to be less than when conventional restorations have been placed (assuming that the bonding process to dentine is not damaging to the pulp!).

Central to the provision of RBMR are techniques to create occlusal space for the restoration; suffice it to say that non-preparation techniques, such as the Dahl approach,[11] involving controlled axial movement of teeth are attractive. In this approach teeth are built-up to cause their intrusion and the supra-eruption of others taken out of occlusion. This topic is summarised in Part 3 of this series. However, it is worth emphasising that the build-up must result in axial loading. Non-axial loading, resulting from a deflective contact or interference on the build-up, can cause problems such as pain and tooth mobility.

In occlusal management
RBMRs are made in the laboratory using the lost wax casting technique. In conjunction with the dental technician, the dentist has good control over form of occlusal surfaces of RBMRs, which can be used therefore to create occlusal stops and guiding surfaces with a high degree of precision. RBMRs are particularly helpful when such teeth are unrestored and where the alternative of conventional crowns would be unacceptably destructive.

A drawback of the technique is that the new guidance surfaces cannot be tested using provisional restorations as with conventional crowns. Guidance surfaces therefore need to be carefully formed with the use of a semi-adjustable articulator and the dentist must accept that some adjustment may be required after the RBMRs have been cemented.

Following molar endodontics
Many posterior teeth which have been root treated are at risk of fracture and will benefit from a protective cusp covering cast restoration.[13] A RBMR with occlusal coverage can provide a conservative restoration for a tooth already compromised by the need for endodontic access.

TECHNIQUES

Choice of metal
If facilities do not exist to heat treat or tin plate gold after try-in, it may be more sensible to use air abraded nickel-chromium, accepting that its shade may look less harmonious in the oral environment than yellow gold.

Design and tooth preparation: anterior teeth
Very thin portions of unsupported buccal enamel remaining on some worn maxillary anterior teeth are highly vulnerable to damage on a stone master cast resulting in a casting which will not fit the tooth. Such enamel should be removed prior to making the impression and defects

waxed-up on the master cast before building up patterns for RBMR (Fig. 3). After cementation, composite resin can be packed against the RBMR to replace lost buccal enamel. The latter technique can also be used to restore pre-existing buccal tooth defects. No other tooth preparation is required for anterior palatal RBMR.

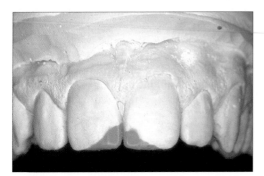

Fig. 3 Enamel defects waxed up on master cast prior to constructing restorations

To optimise adhesion, the maximum possible palatal tooth surface should be covered by the RBMR. Type III gold should probably be a minimum of approximately 0.5 mm thick though it may be reasonable to use nickel-chromium in thinner section because it is more rigid. It is necessary to incorporate features that aid accurate location during seating of the RBMR. A layer of metal overlying the whole of the incisal edge of anterior teeth facilitates accurate seating and following careful thinning can often be left in place without affecting appearance significantly (Fig. 4). In function, the latter feature should also reduce the likelihood that opposing tooth contacts will act directly on the cement layer to cause shear failure.

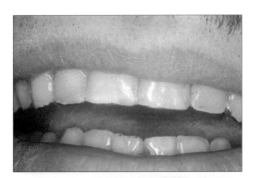

Fig. 4 Appearance of metal incisal coverage because of anterior palatal resin-bonded metal restorations

Design and tooth preparation – posterior teeth

The occlusal part of the restoration must be able to withstand functional forces and, in the absence of evidence to the contrary, dimensions for gold alloy RBMR should follow those recommended for conventional cusp covering crowns (see Part 6). As with anterior RBMRs it may be possible to reduce these dimensions when using nickel-chromium because it is more rigid. Occlusal preparation should only be performed where the treatment plan indicates that occlusal space for the restoration is required (see Part 3).

Table I Precautions for intra-oral air abrasion

Alumina particles are hazardous if inhaled, can scratch glass (eg spectacle lenses) and can leave patients feeling like they have a mouthful of sand. To avoid these problems:

1. Use rubber dam where possible.
2. Pack-off area around tooth with wrung out wet paper towels (alumina will stick to towel – not rebound).
3. Cover patient's whole face including spectacles, with wet paper towels. Fold to allow patient to breathe from beneath towel.
4. Dentist and nurse must wear masks and eye protection.
5. Use high volume aspiration.

Whereas conventional crowns are designed so that non-axial forces tend to put the cement layer in compression (non-adhesive cements are best able to resist compression), RBMR rely substantially on their adhesive luting agent to resist tensile and shearing forces. Axial preparation is useful in as much as it will facilitate accurate orientation on the tooth during bonding. Such a preparation would have an axial reduction of approximately 0.5 mm depth extending down the axial surfaces by one millimetre or so, terminating on a chamfer margin (Fig. 5). Axial preparation will also give the advantage of increasing the surface area for bonding to etched enamel. To what extent axial preparation will help resist peel and shear forces is currently unclear.

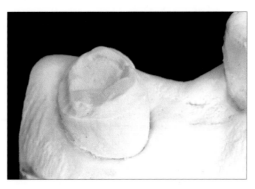

Fig. 5 Preparation form for posterior resin-bonded metal restoration

Managing existing restorations

RBMR rely primarily on adhesion to enamel for retention. Existing restorations which account for a large proportion of the surface area available for adhesion but also extend beyond the periphery of the RBMR are not be ideally suited to restoration using this technique. The critical factor is to finish the margin of the restoration on enamel if at all possible.

Anterior teeth

Restorations deemed to be in need of replacement involving the labial surface of anterior teeth can be managed in several ways:

1. Replace prior to impressions. However by the time the RBMR is cemented the surface will be waterlogged and may only offer sub-optimal bonding to chemically active cements. Use of an intra-oral air abrasion device on the plastic restoration may be beneficial.
2. Remove prior to cementation of RBMR and pack fresh composite against either the trial

seated or cemented RBMR. Placement of composite against the cemented RBMR can make the job of shade matching easier than when replacement is carried out prior to impressions because opaquers and appropriate shades of composite can be used over the metal.

Posterior teeth

Some caution is required in relation to existing restorations that will be completely covered by the RBMR, as they may not offer as great a bond to chemically active cements as etched enamel. Much will therefore depend on the area of enamel available for bonding. Strategies to manage existing restorations, which will be completely covered by the RBMR, would include:

1. Leaving the restoration undisturbed. In this case it may be best to assume that the old restoration offers no additional retention. An example for this approach would be a small sound restoration surrounded by a good periphery of enamel.
2. Air abrading the surface of existing restorations with the aim of providing micromechanical retention for the resin cement (Table 1).
3. Replacement of an existing amalgam restoration with GIC to facilitate bonding.
4. Removal of whole or part of the restoration with the aim of providing a retentive intracoronal feature on the fit surface of the RBMR and exposing tooth structure for bonding. The resulting preparation will resemble that for a conventionally cemented onlay incorporating box forms, bevels and flares.[14] However, removal of old restorations may be associated with unnecessary damage to the tooth and where necessary undercuts should be blocked out with glass ionomer cement.

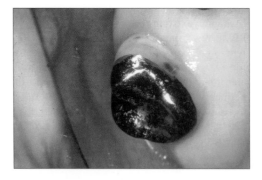

Fig. 6 Appearance of heat-treated gold just after cementation

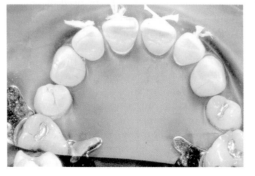

Fig. 7 Floss ligatures to facilitate isolation with rubber dam

Records

Impressions for the laboratory fabrication of RBMR should meet the same quality criteria as for conventional crowns (see Part 10 of this series). Anterior palatal wear often spares a rim of enamel in the proximity of the gingival crevice which should be captured by the impression as it may enhance adhesion significantly. It is helpful to use a gingival retraction technique to achieve this.

Fabrication can be carried out by investing and casting a pattern which has been lifted from the master cast or by forming the pattern for the restoration on refractory material which is itself incorporated within investment.

Bonding

Although occlusal adjustments are more easily polished if carried out before the RBMR is attached to the tooth, stabilising the restoration sufficiently to analyse occlusal contacts can be difficult. A small amount of paraffin jelly smeared onto the fitting surface of the RBMR can provide some retention but needs to be removed completely before bonding.

The fitting surface should ideally be air abraded and steam or ultrasonically cleaned before cementation. Gold alloy RBMR are heat treated at this stage. A brief cycle in a porcelain oven is required (400°C for 4 minutes in air). Despite the colour of the oxidised alloy, no further polishing should be carried out until after the restoration has been cemented as to attempt this risks contaminating the all-important oxide layer developed in the heat treatment (Fig. 6).

In the past there has been concern that the quality of bonding of the chemically active cements advocated for RBMR may be affected by the presence of eugenol.[15] However another study[16] indicates that eugenol containing temporary cements have no adverse effect on the shear bond strength of a dual-curing luting cement to enamel although there may be an effect if a composite core is used.

Several chemically active cements are available to bond RBMR: the same cement as would be chosen for adhesive bridgework. Manufacturers instructions for handling the chosen chemically active cement must be followed closely: it is the responsibility of the dentist to ensure that this is so. Rubber dam is mandatory. Floss ligatures can assist retraction of rubber at the gingival margins of maxillary anterior teeth (Fig. 7). Soft wax on the end of an instrument can be helpful to carry the RBMR to the tooth but great care must be taken not to smear wax onto the fitting surfaces.

After attaching a RBMR to the tooth, removal of excess cement, occlusal adjustments and polishing can be achieved with hand scalers and a sequence of rotary instruments (Table 2). Care must be taken not to overheat the restoration or the resin cement will be softened and the RBMR dislodged.

Table 2 Suggested sequence of instruments for removal of excess set cement at periphery of resin-bonded metal restorations
Hand scalers
Fine and very fine high speed diamond burs
Rubber points
Polishing cup and prophy paste

PROBLEMS

Appearance

Maxillary anterior teeth, which have been thinned by wear on their palatal aspects, may transmit light easily. RBMR luted to the palatal aspects of these teeth may cause a grey colouration that can be unacceptable and is more likely if non-opaque cement is used. On the other hand, opaque cements may help disguise metal but can also cause a lightening in shade. At the initial assessment it is wise to assess possible shade change caused by a RBMR and its cement. White modelling clay applied to the palatal aspect of the thin tooth can mimic the effect of opaque cement. Tin foil burnished onto the palatal surfaces of teeth to be restored can indicate the effect of grey nickel chromium or dark oxidised gold in combination with non-opaque cement.

Showing metal is aesthetically acceptable to some patients but simply not for others! Yellow gold can look more harmonious in the oral environment than nickel-chromium. A useful technique is to use an air abrader to reduce the reflectance of the polished RBMR. In our experience the surface produced by air abrasion also picks up ink of occlusal marking tape more easily than metal left highly polished.[17] A chairside air abrader for intra-oral use is a ideal for this purpose but needs to be used with care (Table 1). The advantages of RBMR should be fully explained to the patient: the informed patient may accept this compromise in appearance.

Temporisation of RBMR

In many cases temporary restorations are unnecessary but as with porcelain labial veneers retention can be a problem. These aspects are addressed in the ninth article in this series.

It is a significant disadvantage that RBMR cannot be reliably attached to teeth for a trial period using temporary cement. Glass ionomer cement (GIC) may afford easy retrieval (or unplanned loss) in some situations but in others acts as a final cement!

MAINTENANCE

Erosion can cause loss of tooth tissue at the periphery of a RBMR (Fig. 8). This problem may occur as a result of not identifying or not controlling the aetiology of the patient's presenting tooth wear. Repair with an adhesive filling material may however be straightforward, although concern has been raised about the ability of the repairing material to bond to the metal casting.

A RBMR whose lute has failed is more likely

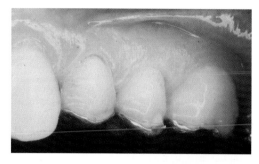

Fig. 8 Recurrent erosion at the periphery of resin-bonded metal restorations *in situ*

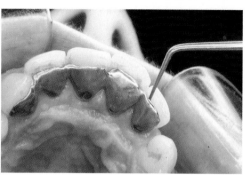

Fig. 9 Partially de-bonded adhesive metal splint

to declare itself by debonding than a conventionally retained crown which may stay in place long enough for the consequences of leakage to take effect. Analysis of the cause of failure for a RBMR may indicate that an attempt should be made to re-attach it after appropriate cleansing and surface treatments. All traces of old cement should be removed from the RBMR, which should then be handled and treated as new. An air abrasion device, abrasive discs and ultrasonic scalers are useful in removing cement from the tooth surface. A round diamond bur can be used without water in a turbine or speed increasing handpiece. The powdery white surface of the instrumented cement can easily be distinguished from the glossy appearance of instrumented enamel. Occasionally etching tooth surface can help to establish whether or not cement remains: areas not appearing frosty are either dentine or residual cement. It is important to remove the resin-infiltrated layer in both enamel and dentine and hence facilitate bonding. Cement removal must be carried out carefully or changes in tooth shape or fit surface of the RBMR will result in an increase in lute thickness. Inevitably, repeated attempts at reattachment are increasingly likely to fail as the lute thickness rises.

RBMRs linked rigidly together to act as a post-orthodontic retainer or periodontal splint, carry the risk that one or more retainers may debond leaving the restoration as a whole attached without causing any initial symptoms. If this happens caries can progress unchecked beneath decemented elements with disastrous results (Fig. 9). Adhesive splints need careful follow-up: patients must be instructed to seek attention if they think a tooth has become debonded. It is often necessary to remove the whole restoration and attempt to re-bond it. A sharp tap to a straight chisel whose blade is positioned at the lute space is often sufficient to dislodge the cemented portions of an adhesive splint. Occasionally it is possible to accept the compromise of removing a decemented retainer if this is at the end of the restoration. Linking RBMR should be avoided wherever possible.

CONCLUSIONS

RBMR rely for their attachment on chemically active cements. The choice is between precious metal and base metal alloys with various surface treatments to enhance adhesion with the cement. RBMR have the potential to be very conservative of tooth tissue but are technique sensitive. To date few clinical studies exist examining their success.

1. Nohl F S, King P A, Harley K E, Ibbetson R J. Retrospective survey of resin-retained cast-metal veneers for the treatment of anterior palatal tooth wear. *Quintessence Int* 1997; **28:** 7-14.
2. Chana H, Kelleher M, Briggs P, Hooper R.J. Clinical evaluation of resin-bonded gold alloy veneers. *J Prosthet Dent* 2000; **83:** 294-300.
3. Foreman P C. Resin-bonded acid-etched onlays in two cases of gross attrition. *Rest Dent* 1988; **15:** 150-153.
4. Harley K E, Ibbetson R J. Dental Anomalies- Are adhesive castings the solution? *Br Dent J* 1993; **174:** 15-22.
5. Lyon H E. Resin-bonded etched-metal rest seats. *J Prosthet Dent* 1985; **53:** 366-368.
6. Thayer K E, Doukoudakis A. Acid-etch canine riser occlusal treatment. *J Prosthet Dent* 1981; **46:** 149-152.
7. Rochette A L. Attachment of a splint to enamel of lower anterior teeth. *J Prosthet Dent* 1973; **30:** 418-423.
8. Livaditis G J, Thompson V P, Etched castings: an improved mechanism for resin bonded retainers. *J Prosthet Dent* 1982; **47:** 52-58.
9. Dixon D L, Breeding L C, Hughie M L, Brown J S. Comparison of shear bond strengths of two resin luting systems for a base and a high noble metal alloy bonded to enamel. *J Prosthet Dent* 1994; **72:** 457-461.
10. Eder A, Wickens J. Surface treatment of gold alloys for resin adhesion. *Quintessence Int* 1996; **27:** 35-40.
11. Hansson O. The Silicoater technique for resin-bonded prostheses: clinical and laboratory procedures. *Quintessence Int* 1989; **20:** 85-99.
12. Dahl B L, Krogstad O, Karlsen K. An alternative treatment in cases with advanced localised attrition. *J Oral Rehabil* 1975: **2:** 209-214.
13. Sorensen J A, Martinoff J T. Intracoronal reinforcement and coronal coverage: a study of endodontically treated teeth. *J Prosthet Dent* 1984; **51:** 780-784.
14. Shillingburg H T, Hobo S, Whitsett L D, Brackett S E. *Fundamentals of fixed prosthodontics*. 3rd ed. pp171-180. Chicago: Quintessence, 1997.
15. Paul S J, Scharer P. Effect of provisional cements on the bond strength of various adhesive systems on dentine. *J Oral Rehabilitation* 1997; **24:** 8-14.
16. Jung M, Gnass C, Senger S. Effect of eugenol-containing temporary cements on bond strength of composite to enamel. *Oper Dent* 1998; **23:** 63-68.
17. Kelleher M G, Setchell D J. An investigation of marking materials used in occlusal adjustment. *Br Dent J* 1984; **156:** 96-102.

Index